EXPANDING ACCESS TO INVESTIGATIONAL THERAPIES FOR HIV INFECTION AND AIDS

March 12-13, 1990
Conference Summary

Eve Nichols

Roundtable for the Development of Drugs
and Vaccines Against AIDS

Institute of Medicine

NATIONAL ACADEMY PRESS
Washington, D.C. 1991

NATIONAL ACADEMY PRESS • 2101 Constitution Avenue, NW • Washington, DC 20418

This conference summary was written by Eve Nichols for the Institute of Medicine's Roundtable for the Development of Drugs and Vaccines Against AIDS, chaired by Harold Ginsberg and Sheldon Wolff and directed by Robin Weiss. The document reports major themes of the conference discussions; these themes, however, do not represent policy statements by the Institute of Medicine.

The report has been reviewed by a group other than the authors according to procedures approved by a Report Review Committee consisting of members of the National Academy of Sciences, the National Academy of Engineering, and the Institute of Medicine.

The Institute of Medicine was chartered in 1970 by the National Academy of Sciences to enlist distinguished members of appropriate professions in the examination of policy matters pertaining to the health of the public. In this, the Institute acts under both the Academy's 1863 congressional charter responsibility to be an advisor to the federal government, and its own initiative in identifying issues of medical care, research, and education.

The Roundtable is supported by the American Foundation for AIDS Research, the Merck Company Foundation, the Pharmaceutical Manufacturers Association, the U.S. Army, the U.S. Public Health Service, and the U.S. Department of Veterans Affairs.

Library of Congress Catalog Card No. 91-60585

International Standard Book Number 0-309-04490-1

Additional copies of this report are available from:

National Academy Press
2101 Constitution Avenue, NW
Washington, DC 20418

S345

Printed in the United States of America

The serpent has been a symbol of long life, healing, and knowledge among almost all cultures and religions since the beginning of recorded history. The image adopted as a logotype by the Institute of Medicine is based on a relief carving from ancient Greece, now held by the Staatlichemuseen in Berlin.

ROUNDTABLE FOR THE DEVELOPMENT OF DRUGS AND VACCINES AGAINST AIDS

HAROLD S. GINSBERG (Co-chair), Eugene Higgins Professor of Medicine and Microbiology, Department of Medicine, College of Physicians & Surgeons, Columbia University, New York

SHELDON M. WOLFF (Co-chair), Physician-in-Chief, New England Medical Center, and Endicott Professor and Chairman, Department of Medicine, Tufts University School of Medicine, Boston

DAVID W. BARRY, Vice President of Research, The Wellcome Research Laboratories, Burroughs Wellcome Co., Research Triangle Park, North Carolina

JAMES S. BENSON, Acting Commissioner, Food and Drug Administration, Rockville, Maryland

DONALD S. BURKE, Colonel, Medical Corps, U.S. Army, and Director, Division of Retrovirology, Walter Reed Army Institute of Research, Rockville, Maryland

BRUCE A. CHABNER, Director, Division of Cancer Treatment, National Cancer Institute, National Institutes of Health, Bethesda, Maryland

MAX D. COOPER, Investigator, Howard Hughes Medical Institute, and Professor of Medicine, Pediatrics, and Microbiology, University of Alabama, Birmingham

MARTIN DELANEY, Co-Executive Director and President, Project Inform, San Francisco

DANIEL DEYKIN, Chief, Cooperative Studies Program, Veterans Administration Medical Center, Boston

R. GORDON DOUGLAS, Senior Vice President, Medical and Scientific Affairs, Merck Sharp & Dohme International, Rahway, New Jersey

ANTHONY S. FAUCI, Associate Director for AIDS Research, National Institutes of Health, and Director, National Institute of Allergy and Infectious Diseases, National Institutes of Health, Bethesda, Maryland

GERALD FRIEDLAND, Professor of Medicine, Department of Medicine, Albert Einstein College of Medicine, Montefiore Medical Center, The Bronx, New York

L. PATRICK GAGE, Executive Vice President, Genetics Institute, Inc., Cambridge, Massachusetts

PETER BARTON HUTT, Partner, Covington & Burling, Washington, D.C.

JAY C. LIPNER, Partner, Silverstein Langer Lipner & Newburgh, New York, New York

DAVID W. MARTIN, JR., Vice President, Research and Development, The Dupont Merck Pharmaceutical Company, Wilmington, Delaware
CATHERINE M. WILFERT, Professor of Pediatrics and Microbiology, Department of Pediatrics, Division of Infectious Diseases, Duke University Medical Center, Durham, North Carolina

STAFF

ROBIN WEISS, Project Director and Director, AIDS Activities
SHARON BARATZ, Research Associate
RICHARD BERZON, Staff Officer
GAIL SPEARS, Administrative Assistant

PREFACE

The Roundtable for the Development of Drugs and Vaccines Against AIDS was established in 1988 by the Institute of Medicine. Composed of leaders from government, the pharmaceutical industry, academia, and the public, its mission is to identify and help resolve impediments to the speedy availability of safe and effective drugs and vaccines for human immunodeficiency virus (HIV) infection and acquired immune deficiency syndrome (AIDS). The Roundtable accomplishes its mission through regular meetings of its membership, during which urgent issues are identified and discussed, as well as through public conferences and workshops that explore scientific and policy matters central to the development of AIDS therapeutics. This publication is the report of a conference held March 12 and 13, 1990, in Washington, D.C.

The call for a "parallel track" for AIDS drug development—a proposal that would allow the early distribution of AIDS drugs to large numbers of patients in parallel with the conventional clinical trials that assess the drugs' safety and efficacy—has sparked controversy within the scientific community. Questions have arisen about the risks to patients of such a plan, about its potential effect on the successful completion of standard controlled trials, and about whether the parallel track will generate useful data. Larger questions have also been raised about whether the parallel track heralds fundamental changes in the philosophy underlying drug regulation in the United States, about the costs and financing of investigational therapies and associated medical costs, and about the role of expanded access mechanisms for drugs in reaching those whose health care generally is inadequate. The Roundtable sought to illuminate these issues by inviting knowledgeable speakers and the public to a two-day conference to examine proposals for expanded access to investigational drugs and possible repercussions of such an action.

Two months after the conference was held, in May 1990, the parallel track proposal was published in the *Federal Register* and comments were sought. A meeting was held in September 1990 by the Public Health Service (PHS) to discuss the comments. As this report goes to press, the PHS is finalizing the document, which, when completed, will constitute a written PHS policy. As the policy takes effect, many of the issues raised in this report will serve as valuable guideposts in evaluating the parallel track experiment.

A note on terminology: Although the word *effectiveness* rather than *efficacy* was used by Congress in the Drug Amendments of 1962, we have chosen in this report to conform to the definitions of the two terms as they are commonly understood in the field of medical technology assessment. Here, the term *efficacy* refers to what a method (e.g., a drug) can accomplish in expert hands when correctly applied to a patient; *effectiveness* refers to its performance in more general routine applications.[1] Therefore, most randomized clinical trials assess efficacy; the Food and Drug Administration, in reviewing the results of these trials, is evaluating the efficacy of the drugs under investigation.

This report seeks to summarize the conference presentations. It contains no recommendations or conclusions, and the Roundtable has neither altered nor commented on the views and opinions expressed by the speakers, except for purposes of clarity. The Roundtable and staff wish to thank Eve Nichols, whose capable hands crafted the transcript of the meeting into a smooth narrative. We also thank, once again, the conference speakers for their thoughtful presentations, and all participants for the lively and challenging discussions throughout the conference.

---

[1]Institute of Medicine, *Assessing Medical Technologies* (Washington, D.C.: National Academy Press, 1985).

CONTENTS

EXPANDING ACCESS TO INVESTIGATIONAL THERAPIES FOR HIV INFECTION AND AIDS

EXPANDING ACCESS TO INVESTIGATIONAL THERAPIES

March 12–13, 1990

PROGRAM

Monday, March 12

8:15 **Welcome and Opening Remarks**
- Harold Ginsberg, Eugene Higgins Professor of Medicine and Microbiology, College of Physicians & Surgeons, Columbia University, and Co-chair, AIDS Roundtable

8:20 **Expanding Access to Investigational Therapies: The Challenges Ahead**
- Samuel O. Thier, President, Institute of Medicine

8:30 **A Lucid Explanation and Brief History of Food and Drug Administration Policy on Investigational Drugs for Treatment Purposes**
- Peter Barton Hutt, Partner, Covington & Burling

9:00 **The Promise of Treatment Investigational New Drug Regulations: Have They Done What They Were Supposed to Do?**

Moderator:
J. Richard Crout, Vice President, Medical and Scientific Affairs, Boehringer Mannheim Pharmaceuticals

Panelists:
Robert Temple, Director, Office of Drug Evaluation I, Food and Drug Administration
Jay Lipner, Partner, Silverstein Langer Lipner & Newburgh
Stephen Sherwin, Vice President for Clinical Research, Genentech, Inc.

1

Lawrence Corey, Professor of Laboratory Medicine, Micro-
biology, and Medicine, University of Washington
Raphael Dolin, Head, Infectious Diseases Unit, University of
Rochester School of Medicine and Dentistry

10:00   **Discussion**

10:45   **The Philosophy of Drug Regulation in the United States: Is It
Changing from Beneficence to Patient Autonomy?**

Moderator:
Dan Brock, Professor of Philosophy, Brown University

Panelists:
Harold Edgar, Professor of Law, Columbia University School
of Law
Bernard Lo, Director, Program in Medical Ethics, University
of California
Daniel Wikler, Professor, Department of Philosophy, Univer-
sity of Wisconsin
Carol Levine, Executive Director, Citizens Commission on
AIDS

12:00   **Discussion**

1:45   **Issues of Cost and Coverage: How Will the Changes Affect the
Drug Industry, Payers, and Patients?**

Moderator:
Patrick Gage, Executive Vice President, Genetics Institute,
Inc.

Panelists:
Jerome Birnbaum, Executive Vice President for Research,
Bristol-Myers Squibb Company
Paul De Stefano, Chief Corporate Counsel, Genentech, Inc.
David Higbee, Branch Chief, Catastrophic Medical Services,
Office of Coverage Policy, Health Care Financing Adminis-
tration
Susan Gleeson, Executive Director, Technology Management,
Blue Cross and Blue Shield Association
Steven Peskin, Vice President and Medical Director, CIGNA
Healthplan of Texas, Inc.

Lee Mortenson, Executive Director, Association of
Community Cancer Centers

3:00   **Discussion**

3:45   **Expanding Access and Gathering and Analyzing Data: Can You
        Have Your Cake and Eat It Too?**

Moderator:
Lincoln Moses, Professor of Statistics, Stanford University

Panelists:
Melanie Thompson, President, AIDS Research Consortium of
    Atlanta, Inc.
Marvin Zelen, Chair, Department of Biostatistics, Harvard
    School of Public Health
Floyd J. Fowler, Senior Research Fellow, Center for Survey
    Research, University of Massachusetts
Susan Ellenberg, Chief, Biostatistics Research Branch, Divi-
    sion of AIDS, National Institute of Allergy and Infectious
    Diseases

5:00   **Discussion**

5:30   **Adjournment**

Tuesday, March 13

8:15   **Reaching the Disenfranchised: What Role for Clinical Trials?**

Moderator:
Gerald Friedland, Professor of Medicine, Epidemiology, and
    Social Medicine, Albert Einstein College of Medicine

Panelists:
Lawrence Brown, Jr., Senior Vice President for Research and
    Medical Affairs, Addiction Research and Treatment Cor-
    poration
Mark Smith, Associate Director, AIDS Service, Johns Hop-
    kins University School of Medicine
Deborah Cotton, Clinical Director for AIDS, Beth Israel
    Hospital

Philip Pizzo, Chief, Pediatric Branch, National Cancer
Institute

9:30   **Discussion**

10:15   **Parallel Track: An Update**
        – James Allen, Director, National AIDS Program Office, Public
          Health Service

10:30   **Parallel Track: What Should It Achieve?**

        Moderator:
            Anthony Fauci, Associate Director for AIDS Research, Na-
            tional Institutes of Health, and Director, National Institute
            of Allergy and Infectious Diseases

        Panelists:
            Louis Lasagna, Dean, Sackler School of Graduate Biomedi-
            cal Sciences, Tufts University
            James Eigo, Member, Treatment and Data Committee, AIDS
            Coalition to Unleash Power
            Daniel Hoth, Director, Division of AIDS, National Institute
            of Allergy and Infectious Diseases
            Ellen Cooper, Director, Division of Antiviral Drug Products,
            Food and Drug Administration

11:45   **Discussion**

12:15   **Expanding Access and the Needs of the Traditional Primary
        Care Provider**
        – Harvey Makadon, Assistant Professor of Medicine, Harvard
          Medical School, and Executive Director, Boston AIDS
          Consortium

12:35   **Discussion**

12:50   **Summation**
        – Sheldon Wolff, Endicott Professor and Chairman, Department
          of Medicine, Tufts University School of Medicine, and Co-
          chair, AIDS Roundtable

1:00   **Adjournment**

1

HISTORICAL PERSPECTIVE

In the second week of March 1990, headlines across the country described an unusual scientific controversy over the distribution of an investigational drug called dideoxyinosine (ddI) to thousands of patients with acquired immune deficiency syndrome (AIDS). Newspapers reported that patients receiving the drug through a new expanded access program had a much higher death rate than patients enrolled in conventional clinical trials of the drug.   In one case, a Harvard faculty member was quoted as saying that death rates in the expanded access program were "a disgrace, an absolute disgrace."   But many physicians advised their HIV (human immunodeficiency virus)-infected patients to keep taking the drug.   Officials at the Food and Drug Administration (FDA), advocates for people with AIDS, and the drug's sponsor, Bristol-Myers Squibb, attributed most or even all of the disparity in death rates to the fact that patients enrolled in the expanded access program were sicker to begin with than those in the clinical trials.

The ddI controversy exposed sharp differences of opinion within the medical community about the appropriateness of making investigational drugs—drugs not yet approved for marketing by the FDA—available for therapeutic purposes. In August 1989, the Public Health Service (PHS) convened a committee to formalize procedures for making promising investigational agents available to people with AIDS and other HIV-related disorders who could not participate in controlled clinical trials and who had no therapeutic alternatives. The committee's recommendations were still in draft form seven months later,

This chapter is based primarily on the presentation of Peter Barton Hutt.   Other contributors include Jay Lipner, Lawrence Corey, James Allen, Louis Lasagna, James Eigo, Daniel Hoth, and Ellen Cooper.

but many people regarded the ddI trial as the prototype of the new "parallel track system." (On May 21, 1990, the Department of Health and Human Services published a proposed policy statement, "Expanded Availability of Investigational New Drugs Through a Parallel Track Mechanism for People with AIDS and HIV-related Disease," in the *Federal Register.*)

The controversy continues today. Opponents of the parallel track worry that it will disrupt efforts to assess the safety and efficacy of drug candidates through conventional clinical trials. They question the value of information gathered through the parallel track system and express concern about exposing large numbers of people to relatively unknown agents. Advocates of parallel track acknowledge that increasing access to investigational drugs without definitive evidence of either safety or efficacy carries serious potential risks, but they believe that many desperately ill patients are willing to assume such risks. After all, they say, investigational drugs are the only hope for thousands of AIDS patients who either cannot tolerate or fail to respond to zidovudine (commonly known as AZT), the only anti-HIV drug licensed in the United States.

One fact often ignored by both sides is that access to investigational drugs for therapeutic purposes is not new in this country. In fact, it is as old as the history of drug regulation itself. Two features that make the current situation somewhat different from the past are (1) the desire to establish a written policy and (2) the large number of people who could receive a single investigational drug in a short period of time. A brief review of earlier approaches to expanded access and a summary of the drug approval process prior to the start of the AIDS epidemic help place the debate over the parallel track mechanism in perspective.

EARLY DEVELOPMENT OF EXPANDED ACCESS

Modern drug regulation in the United States began in 1938 with enactment of the Federal Food, Drug, and Cosmetic Act, prompted by the elixir sulfanilamide tragedy of November 1937 (more than 100 people died when a drug containing the poisonous solvent diethylene glycol was marketed without animal tests). The new act contained one brief section, labeled 505(i), in which Congress authorized the FDA to issue rules governing investigational use of drug candidates. The FDA regulations that resulted from this authorization contained four requirements: (1) an experimental drug had to be labeled "for investigational use only"; (2) the drug could be delivered only to experts and could be used by them solely for investigational purposes; (3) each expert had to have adequate facilities for investigation; and (4) the sponsor had to have a signed statement from the investigator indicating that the drug would be used solely for investigational purposes until it had been fully licensed.

The regulations did not describe "expert" qualifications or specify the nature of "adequate facilities." In fact, they did not even define "investigational use." Thus, in practice, the sponsor could provide an investigational drug to any physician who was willing to sign the required statement. Questions of expanded access did not arise because there were no substantive barriers to obtaining investigational drugs for therapeutic purposes.

Drug Amendments of 1962

Public attention did not focus again on the drug regulatory apparatus until July 1962, when a story in the *Washington Post* disclosed links between the experimental drug thalidomide and severe birth defects. Three months later, the U.S. Congress unanimously passed the first major drug amendments.

Surprisingly, the 1962 amendments did not radically alter section 505(i). They authorized regulations for investigational new drugs but did not require the submission of study plans, record keeping, or statements from investigators. The only mandatory provision was that investigators had to obtain informed consent from every subject.

The regulations issued by the FDA in response to the thalidomide tragedy and the new statute provided the first formal structure for the drug development process. Before beginning clinical trials, all sponsors would have to submit an investigational new drug application, or IND. The IND would describe the chemical structure of the new compound and its probable mode of action in the body, identify investigators, describe the results of laboratory and animal tests, and outline specific elements of the study protocol.

Access for Therapeutic Purposes

The FDA press release that accompanied the final regulations in January 1963 addressed for the first time the issue of access to investigational drugs for therapeutic purposes. In an analysis of objections that had been raised to the regulations in draft form, the press release noted, "The proposed regulations were said to deny extremely important new drugs not yet approved for general distribution to patients who might need them urgently as a lifesaving measure."

The FDA's response set the tone for the next two decades. The press release explained, "The increased flexibility in the regulations will allow the sponsor of a new drug investigation to add new investigators after the program is started. There is no bar in the regulations to giving the necessary instructions to, and obtaining the necessary commitments from, a new investigator by telephone in case this is needed to save a life."

Growing Confusion

From 1962 until the beginning of the 1980s, access to investigational drugs was an informal process governed primarily by telephone. The FDA had no written policies. If a physician determined that a severely ill patient had no recourse other than an experimental drug, the physician called the FDA and requested access to that drug. Medical officers in the agency evaluated each situation separately and either approved or denied the request. The criteria were simple. Approval required four basic elements: a manufacturer willing to supply the drug, a physician willing to prescribe it, a patient willing to give informed consent, and some basis for believing that the treatment was not an outright fraud or poison.

The flexibility of this system enabled many very sick patients to receive drugs with a minimum of delay and paperwork. But there were also drawbacks to the informal approach. First, the system only worked for patients whose physicians knew what drugs were under investigation; patients treated by physicians outside the mainstream of academic medicine were less likely to have access to experimental therapies. Second, some ineffective or even toxic drugs, such as DMSO (dimethyl sulfoxide), attained widespread distribution among patients whose original illnesses did not justify extreme measures. Finally, the lack of written policies spawned a confusing array of terms and concepts that still cloud discussions and interfere with efforts to develop a more uniform approach to the access problem.

In the 1960s, FDA medical officers permitted access to investigational drugs under several mechanisms: orphan drug INDs, individual investigator INDs, and compassionate use INDs. The orphan drug concept actually predated the 1962 amendments and remains in use today. It refers to drugs developed to treat rare or unusual conditions. The "permanent" orphan drug IND was conceived to provide access to drugs that would never meet licensure requirements because there were simply too few patients to collect adequate data. (In 1983, Congress passed the Orphan Drug Act to provide certain tax and other financial incentives to the sponsors of therapies for rare diseases.)

The individual investigator IND enabled physicians to obtain experimental drugs for therapeutic purposes when it was not possible to enroll their patients in existing clinical trials. By the end of the 1960s, this concept had been incorporated into the compassionate use IND, which also covered the provision of experimental drugs to patients during FDA review of a new drug application, or NDA (the document submitted by a sponsor after the completion of clinical trials to request permission for marketing).

Two more expanded access concepts arose during the 1970s. Sponsors of controlled trials were permitted to develop concurrent open-label safety studies (also called open enrollment or open protocol). Through these studies, which continue today, thousands of patients received access to experimental drugs at various stages of investigation. Although the FDA requires sponsors of these studies to collect safety data, many observers of FDA policy believe that the primary purpose of the open-label studies is to provide therapy to patients. In 1976, the FDA also accepted the concept of the Group C cancer drug IND, which provides increased access to certain investigational cancer drugs distributed by the National Cancer Institute.

It is important to remember that all of these concepts evolved in the absence of any written policy. Over the years, several groups in Congress and the FDA attempted to develop a more rational approach to the use of investigational drugs for therapeutic purposes, but changes in administration and other political events intervened. Meanwhile, the drug development and approval process itself grew increasingly formal. By 1980, it took an average of 10 years for a new drug to progress from the laboratory to the medicine chest.

Modern Clinical Trials (Non-AIDS Drugs)

With some important exceptions, the basic framework of the drug evaluation process today is similar to that of 10 years ago (although a study by the Pharmaceutical Manufacturers Association suggests that the average time to FDA approval now may be closer to 12 years). If preclinical investigations indicate that a drug has biological activity against a targeted disease and does not cause unacceptable damage to healthy tissues, the drug sponsor requests permission from the FDA to begin the first of three phases of clinical trials—that is, the sponsor files an IND.

Phase 1 studies usually take a year and may involve up to 50 normal, healthy volunteers. These are short-term tolerance and clinical pharmacology studies; their goals are to begin to establish the drug's safety in human beings and to determine appropriate dose levels and routes of administration. (Phase 1 studies of drugs for life-threatening conditions, such as AIDS and cancer, or of drugs that are very toxic may involve patients with the target disease rather than healthy volunteers. Patient studies are also preferred when investigators shorten preclinical studies to speed drug development. As a result of the shortened preclinical studies, the potential for toxicity may be too great to justify giving the drug to someone who has no chance of benefiting from it.)

Phase 2 trials, which usually take two years or more, involve 100 to 300 consenting patients. Investigators gather additional information about possible adverse effects and begin to assess a drug's clinical potential. Most phase 2 studies are randomized, controlled trials. A group of patients receiving the drug, a "treatment" group, is matched with a group that is similar in important respects, such as age, gender, and disease state (factors that could affect the course of the disease or the effect of the investigational drug). The second, or "control," group receives another treatment such as standard therapy or a placebo (an inert substance). Many phase 2 studies are double blind—that is, neither the patient nor the researchers know who is getting the experimental drug. The purpose of double-blind studies is to reduce errors in interpretation caused by unwarranted enthusiasm or other forms of bias.

Phase 3 clinical trials involve many more volunteer patients—several hundred to several thousand—and last about three years. The larger trials allow researchers to acquire more information about efficacy and to identify some of the less common side effects associated with an experimental drug.

If the net results of all three phases of clinical trials are favorable and the sponsor decides to market the drug, it submits a new drug application to the FDA. The NDA must contain all the scientific information gathered in the previous years and typically runs 100,000 pages or more. The average time between the submission of an NDA and final FDA approval is close to three years.

THE ADVENT OF AIDS

The AIDS epidemic has drawn unprecedented attention to the entire drug approval process and prompted or accelerated a variety of changes—some of which were under consideration before the epidemic began. These changes fall into three categories: efforts to broaden patient and community involvement in developing and testing new products, efforts to shorten the overall development and review process, and efforts to increase access to promising drugs before FDA approval (expanded access).

Broadening Participation

Throughout most of the 1980s, people with AIDS and their advocates were highly critical of the FDA and other government agencies involved in drug development. There was a perception that government scientists were more interested in maintaining the scientific standards of clinical trials than in providing new options for the thousands of patients who were dying as a result of HIV infection. Government scientists, on the other hand, were frustrated by misconceptions surrounding the drug development process. For example, the role of the FDA is to ensure that drugs marketed in the United States meet established standards of safety and efficacy; the FDA could not initiate or conduct clinical trials on its own, as some patient advocates were suggesting.

Over time, the adversarial relationship has relaxed somewhat, although strong disagreements remain. Persons with AIDS and their advocates now participate on advisory committees within the Public Health Service to provide practical advice about the optimal design and implementation of clinical trials from the patient's perspective. In addition, scientists at the helm of the research effort in AIDS have recognized the need for creative approaches to the problems associated with HIV infection.

One result of this cooperation was the establishment in October 1989 of a new AIDS treatment research initiative called Community Programs for Clinical Research on AIDS (CPCRA), funded by the National Institute of Allergy and Infectious Diseases (NIAID). Before the advent of CPCRA, all federally funded clinical trials of experimental AIDS drugs were conducted by investigators at the National Institutes of Health or at the 47 university-based research hospitals associated with the AIDS Clinical Trials Group (ACTG). (Of course, pharmaceutical companies and community-based physicians have also conducted important clinical trials of AIDS drugs.) The ACTG consortium was created by NIAID in 1986 to perform the complex multidisciplinary clinical and laboratory studies required for development of new antiviral drugs.

Although AIDS activists and community care providers recognized the contributions made by ACTG investigators, they questioned the need to restrict federally funded clinical trials to university medical centers. They claimed that many important research and clinical questions could be addressed in settings that lacked the technological sophistication of the ACTG institutions. Also, demographic information on patients in ACTG studies revealed that, although some of the large medical centers are also inner-city hospitals that treat underserved patient populations, other ACTUs (AIDS clinical trial units) were not reaching certain patient groups. (Underserved populations have included people of color, women, and intravenous drug users infected with HIV.) As a result, these groups did not have access to potentially beneficial investigational drugs.

CPCRA was designed to address these issues. The 18 diverse CPCRA sites give community care providers and their HIV-infected patients opportunities to participate in clinical trials. The program is designed to take advantage of the clinical expertise acquired by physicians in private practice, in community clinics, and at larger inner-city hospitals. In addition, NIAID seeks, through these new sites, to increase access for underserved populations to experimental therapies. As noted in Chapter 7, however, much more work remains to be done to solve the access problem.

Accelerating the Pace of Drug Development

One of the hardest messages to convey to desperately ill patients has been that no changes in regulations or clinical trials can increase access to drugs unless potential drug candidates are already in the pipeline. Historically, medical science has not fared well in the battle against chronic viral infections such as herpes, hepatitis B, cytomegalovirus, and AIDS. The successes against HIV infection—represented by zidovudine, and perhaps ddI—have resulted from very recent advances in virology, cell culture, and molecular biology.

In 1986, NIAID started the National Cooperative Drug Discovery Group to stimulate new research on targeted development of AIDS drugs. The group's efforts have complemented work by the Preclinical AIDS Drug Development Program at the National Cancer Institute, which screens thousands of natural and synthetic compounds each year for activity against HIV. As of January 1990, the FDA had granted permission for IND studies involving more than 80 different AIDS-related antiviral or immunomodulating drugs. Experience suggests, however, that fewer than 20 percent of these will survive the trials and approval process.

Improving Response Capabilities

Recognizing that FDA would be called upon to respond rapidly to the new challenges posed by AIDS, then commissioner Frank E. Young made a number of administrative and organizational changes at the agency. First, he assigned all AIDS treatments a special 1-AA designation, giving them top review priority. This meant that the FDA intended to act on all AIDS-related NDAs within 180 days of their submission. A new division of antiviral drug products was created within FDA's Center for Biologics Evaluation and Research to expedite the review and evaluation of potential AIDS therapies. In addition, FDA established the AIDS Coordination Staff to integrate the agency's various AIDS-related activities and to interact with other agencies and outside groups interested in AIDS drug development.

Expedited Development

Perhaps the most fundamental change, however, involved the clinical trials process itself. In October 1988, Dr. Young announced immediate implementation of a formal plan to reduce the time required for human testing of drugs for life-threatening and severely debilitating diseases, such as AIDS, Parkinson's disease, and certain aggressive cancers. The primary effect of the new "expedited development" process is to eliminate phase 3 clinical trials for drugs shown to improve survival or prevent irreversible morbidity. By planning the critical phase 2 studies well, the development and review process might be shortened by two to three years.

Expedited development follows a pattern established by the development of zidovudine. In February 1986, after a promising phase 1 trial at the National Cancer Institute and Duke University, researchers started a phase 2 study of zidovudine at 12 medical centers across the United States (the placebo-controlled randomized trial involved patients with AIDS or advanced AIDS-related complex [ARC]). The phase 2 study was stopped in September of that year, when an independent data safety monitoring board found a dramatic difference in outcomes between the 145 patients receiving zidovudine and the 137 patients receiving placebos (19 patients in the placebo arm of the trial had died, compared with only a single death in the zidovudine group). Burroughs Wellcome, the manufacturer, submitted a new drug application for zidovudine in December 1986. The FDA approved the NDA without a phase 3 clinical trial on March 20, 1987. At the time, officials explained that one reason for the rapid approval of zidovudine was that FDA scientists had had an opportunity to work closely with the drug's sponsor from the very beginning of the development process.

Current procedures for expedited development specify that the FDA will meet with drug sponsors to help devise efficient animal and human studies—studies that answer vital questions about safety and efficacy in the least amount of time possible. The FDA also monitors the progress of clinical trials and, if necessary, helps the sponsor develop appropriate postmarketing studies to provide additional information about risks, benefits, optimal uses, and dosages. The FDA approval process for drugs in the expedited pathway takes into consideration the severity of the disease being treated and the availability of alternative therapies, as well as the statutory criteria for approval.

Expanded Access

The urgency created by the AIDS epidemic also has focused attention on two approaches to expanded access: the treatment IND and the parallel track protocol. These mechanisms, which incorporate the expanded use practices that began in the 1960s, evolved from a growing awareness on the part of drug sponsors, government scientists, and others that the informal procedures of the past would not be sufficient to handle the distribution of investigational drugs to AIDS patients. The complexity of HIV infection and the potential toxicity of some drug candidates discouraged FDA medical officers from approving expanded access protocols for AIDS drugs on the basis of a few quick telephone conversations. There also was concern that the volume of requests might become overwhelming.

Treatment Investigational New Drugs

The treatment IND first emerged as part of a long-term effort to incorporate the concept of expanded access into the IND regulations.

In June 1983, the FDA issued proposed regulations that included a very broad interpretation of the use of investigational drugs for therapeutic purposes: at any time during the investigational process, the FDA could approve a treatment protocol for any patient with a serious disease (the definition of "serious" was left to the discretion of the patient and physician). The proposed interpretation would have incorporated virtually all of the older versions of expanded access, including the compassionate use IND and the orphan drug IND.

Some critics believe that when the final IND regulations emerged in 1987, the definition of treatment IND was much narrower. The treatment IND mechanism allows patients suffering from serious or life-threatening conditions for which there is no satisfactory alternative therapy to obtain a promising experimental drug. Clinical evidence must be available to show that the drug is relatively safe and that it "may be effective." In addition, controlled clinical trials must be completed or ongoing and the sponsor must be pursuing marketing with "due diligence." Others at the FDA argue that the only real difference between the 1983 and 1987 versions of the regulations was that the 1987 announcement received a great deal of publicity, which reminded the public that the treatment IND was an available mechanism.

A government scientist reports that, as of March 12, 1990, the FDA had approved 18 treatment INDs for conditions ranging from AIDS to respiratory distress syndrome in infants. Almost 20,000 patients had obtained access to drugs not yet approved for marketing. Nevertheless, persons with AIDS and their advocates say that the treatment IND has fallen far short of their expectations. They suggest that the FDA's interpretation and implementation of "may be effective" have been too rigorous—too close to the standard used for final approval of a drug. With one exception, they say, treatment INDs have simply bridged the gap between the end of clinical trials and full FDA approval. They have not increased access to drugs at earlier stages of development or helped patients who were ineligible for conventional clinical trials.

Another criticism of the treatment IND regulations has been that they increased, rather than decreased, confusion about the parameters of expanded access. People inside and outside the government had hoped that the regulations would furnish a framework for all of the different approaches to providing experimental drugs to desperately ill patients. Instead, the regulations defined one particularly narrow approach and left other options open. Early dissatisfaction with the treatment IND led to calls for a more flexible solution to the access problem.

Parallel Track

For almost a year after the release of the new IND regulations, patient advocates, community physicians, and government scientists exchanged ideas about other possible ways to expand access to experimental drugs. Finally, at a meeting in San Francisco in June 1989, Anthony Fauci, director of the National Institute of Allergy and Infectious Diseases, presented the concept of the "parallel track" protocol. The parallel track would make selected drugs available to HIV-infected patients who could not participate in conventional clinical trials and who had no therapeutic alternatives, without disrupting the progress of controlled clinical trials. Parallel track protocols could be approved for promising investigational drugs when the evidence for effectiveness was less than that required for a treatment IND.

Several months later, an FDA Advisory Committee meeting convened by the FDA and a subgroup convened by the National AIDS Program Office began efforts to define the structure of the parallel track system. After a lengthy review process, they decided that parallel track protocols could be implemented within the framework of existing regulations. In December 1989, they submitted a proposed policy statement explaining the basic outlines of the parallel track to the Office of the Secretary of Health and Human Services. Drugs would be considered for the new track only if manufacturers could provide the following:

1. information showing promising evidence of efficacy based on an assessment of all available laboratory and clinical data, as well as sufficient information to recommend an appropriate starting dose and preliminary pharmacokinetic and dose-response data;
2. evidence that the investigational drug is reasonably safe, taking into consideration the intended use and the prospective patient population;
3. a description of the intended patient population;
4. evidence that the defined patient population lacks satisfactory alternative therapies;
5. assurance that the manufacturer is willing and able to produce sufficient quantities of the drug for both controlled clinical trials and the parallel track;

6. a statement of the status of existing controlled clinical trial protocols (drugs will be considered for parallel track only after protocols for phase 2 controlled clinical trials have been approved by the FDA; also, patient enrollment in phase 2 controlled trials must start before or concurrently with the release of drugs for parallel track);

7. an assessment of the impact that the parallel track study may have on patient enrollment in controlled clinical trials and a proposed plan for monitoring progress of the controlled trials; and

8. information describing the educational efforts that will be undertaken by the manufacturer or the sponsor to ensure that participating physicians and potential recipients have sufficient knowledge of the potential risks and benefits of the investigational agent.

Evidence for safety and efficacy might come in part from expanded phase 1 trials. As noted earlier, phase 1 trials for drugs for AIDS and other life-threatening diseases often involve persons with the disease instead of healthy volunteers. The expedited development process and the potential increase in the number of people who might get very early access to an experimental drug for therapeutic purposes have placed pressure on investigators to get as much information as possible from phase 1 trials. For example, the authors of the proposed policy statement on the parallel track indicate that expanded phase 1 trials should provide some information about potential interactions between an investigational drug and other drugs commonly used in the patient population. Other physicians suggest that expanded phase 1 trials should compare different doses of an experimental drug, primarily to avoid problems similar to those that arose with zidovudine. (Two years after the FDA approved zidovudine, a randomized trial carried out by the ACTG revealed that patients taking 600 milligrams per day of the drug did as well as patients taking the recommended dose of 1.2 grams per day. If this had been known sooner, some patients might have avoided adverse reactions, and many more would have been spared unnecessary expense.)

The proposed policy statement on parallel track also outlines eligibility requirements for patients. First, patients must have clinically significant HIV-related illness or be at imminent health risk as a result of HIV-related immunodeficiency. Second, patients must be unable to participate in related controlled clinical trials, either because they do not meet entry criteria (for example, laboratory test results are not within specified limits), because they are too sick, or because participation would create undue hardship (the nature of possible hardships, such as travel time to a research center, must be described in the parallel track protocol). Finally, physicians who wish to enroll a patient in the parallel track must provide evidence that existing FDA-approved therapies for the condition are contraindicated for that patient, that the patient cannot tolerate them, or that they are no longer effective.

Close monitoring of the parallel track will be essential to ensure that serious adverse effects (or, conversely, unexpected benefits) are recognized at the earliest possible moment. According to the proposed policy statement, sponsors will be required to establish a data and safety monitoring board (DSMB) with responsibility for overseeing the parallel track protocol and for comparing information gathered from the parallel track with information gathered from related clinical trials. The recent experience with ddI, described at the beginning of this chapter, underscores the importance of reviewing all available materials. Although data collection in the parallel track will be minimal compared with data collection in controlled trials, the DSMB should have a sufficient basis for comparison. If necessary, the DSMB or its equivalent may recommend to the FDA, to the sponsor, or to the NIAID AIDS Research Advisory Committee that the parallel track protocol—and possibly related clinical trials—be terminated.

In conventional clinical trials, educational materials and informed consent documents that describe the potential risks and benefits associated with an experimental drug must be approved by an institutional review board (IRB) at each participating institution. The PHS working group, however, determined that such an arrangement might be impractical for parallel track protocols, in part because many community physicians who wished to participate in the parallel track would not have access to IRBs. In addition, the time required to provide sufficient information to hundreds of IRBs around the country would defeat the main purpose of the parallel track—rapid dissemination of investigational drugs to desperately ill patients.

To overcome this problem, the working group has proposed a national human subjects protection review panel to provide continuing ethical oversight of all parallel track protocols. The panel would have a diverse membership, including persons with AIDS, physicians, government scientists, and others. It would be responsible for establishing the types of information that must be given to patients and for approving all informed consent procedures.

2

RIGHTS AND RESPONSIBILITIES

The philosophical debate over expanded access to investigational drugs takes many forms. People often try to reduce the standard arguments to simple dichotomies; for example, the "mind versus heart" approach pits the scientific discipline of clinical trials against the compassionate use of experimental drugs for therapeutic purposes. The "beneficence versus autonomy" approach suggests that providing protection to people with HIV infection must conflict with respect for their individual rights.

In fact, most efforts to simplify the debate over expanded access do a disservice by diverting attention from a host of complex issues that must be considered in any discussion of increased access to AIDS drugs. These issues concern (1) the need for constraints on freedom of choice, (2) the capacity for informed consent in an environment characterized by restricted access to health care, (3) the potential for setting the rights of today's patients against the rights of future patients, (4) the shifts in concerns of institutional review boards, and (5) the problems that could arise from early and close collaboration between the FDA and drug sponsors.

FREEDOM OF CHOICE

The expedited review process, treatment IND regulations, and recent efforts to establish a parallel track system for AIDS drugs (all described in Chapter 1) have led some people to suggest that the FDA is moving away from its traditional role of consumer protection

---

This chapter is based on the presentations of J. Richard Crout, Dan Brock, Harold Edgar, Bernard Lo, Daniel Wikler, and Carol Levine.

toward a new vision of patient autonomy. Scientists involved in these programs indicate, however, that they were never intended to promote freedom of choice as an independent value in drug development. Instead, they were designed to increase options for desperately ill patients with no therapeutic alternatives.

The extreme argument for freedom of choice has been that persons infected with HIV have "little or nothing to lose," so why limit their access to any drugs? The problem with this argument is that it fails to recognize the association between desperation and vulnerability. Exploitation of people with HIV infection by unscrupulous vendors with worthless products has been a significant problem. People with HIV infection do have something to lose: they can waste time, energy, and hope—or even become sicker—on substances that would never reach the marketplace through normal channels.

Totally free access to substances that may or may not be fraudulent is quite different from the opportunity to make informed, reasoned choices about products for which there is a reasonable expectation of effectiveness (based on preclinical or early clinical data). Clearly, persons with life-threatening illnesses are willing to assume greater risks in exchange for smaller potential benefits than other groups of patients. Expanded access programs recognize the right to assume such risks—with the advice and assistance of a personal physician—without abandoning the individual to the forces of the marketplace.

INFORMED CONSENT

Early experiences with both treatment INDs and the parallel track approach have demonstrated that several external factors can limit a person's ability to make informed, reasoned choices about participation in experimental protocols. Two of the most troublesome factors are the lack of adequate information about drug products and the shortage of health care options—for some people with HIV disease, clinical trials may represent the only opportunity for access to a knowledgeable medical team.

Information Resources

For most persons with HIV infection and their physicians, the first encounter with a new drug or treatment alternative occurs through the lay press. Traditional attitudes within the medical establishment about publishing first in the medical literature and then in the press have been tempered with regard to AIDS because of the recognized need to get information out "on the streets" as quickly as possible. News about successful studies fosters hope and gives patients a sense of control that they might not otherwise have.

But there are also disadvantages to this strategy. Physicians who treat HIV-infected patients complain that news reports do not have sufficient clinical detail to allow them or their patients to make informed decisions. For example, the patient may be especially concerned about one particular side effect of a drug, such as fatigue. News reports rarely present specific information about the incidence of an adverse effect unless the problem is severely debilitating.

The long delay between publicity about a new therapy and the publication of peer-reviewed journal articles limits the physician's ability to add substance to the decisionmaking process. Events surrounding the establishment of a treatment IND for aerosolized pentamidine illustrate this concern. The treatment IND was issued in February 1989, simultaneously with a press release announcing the effectiveness of the therapy as prophylaxis for *Pneumocystis carinii* pneumonia. San Francisco investigators presented a formal abstract describing community trials of the treatment at the international AIDS meeting in Montreal several months later, and by late June the FDA had approved the drug for marketing. As of March 1990, however, data from the community trial of aerosolized pentamidine still had not been published in a peer-reviewed journal.[1]

Another problem with depending on the media to disseminate information is the potential for bias. Reporters may have difficulty achieving objectivity in a news report based on a press conference called by a drug manufacturer, a funding agency, or an investigator who has devoted several years to a drug study. The need for eye-catching headlines also hinders efforts to place new discoveries in perspective.

Physicians who treat HIV-infected patients have suggested several ways to improve communication about promising new drugs. One suggestion has been to encourage a standard format for press releases

---

[1]Results of this trial appeared in G. S. Leoung, D. W. Feigal, A. B. Montgomery, D. Corkery, L. Wardlaw, M. Adams, D. Busch, S. Gordon, M. A. Jacobson, P. A. Volberding, D. Abrams, and the San Francisco County Community Consortium, "Aerosolized pentamidine for prophylaxis against *Pneumocystis carinii* pneumonia: The San Francisco Community Prophylaxis Trial," *New England Journal of Medicine*, vol. 323, no. 12, pp. 769–775 (1990).

that includes basic information about study subjects, methodology, end-points, and results (the same type of information that would be included in a formal abstract). Another option is to speed up journal publication. Alternatively, an independent group could be designated to review data and present key results in an informational letter to physicians, perhaps in the *FDA Drug Bulletin*. Other options include a mechanism similar to the "Clinical Alert System" adopted by the National Cancer Institute, or a federally sponsored on-line data base that would provide relevant data from clinical trials to HIV-infected patients and their physicians.

The proposed policy statement for parallel track protocols emphasizes the development of appropriate mechanisms to educate potential drug recipients and their physicians. Initially, the sponsor must provide patients with enough information to compare the potential risks and benefits of a new drug with the risks and benefits of other treatment options. The sponsor also has the more difficult task of ensuring that information acquired during the course of a parallel track protocol—especially with regard to adverse effects—is relayed to participants as quickly as possible. Physicians involved in the early days of the parallel track protocol for ddI report that lack of such information sometimes hampered their efforts to provide appropriate care for their patients.

Access

Two different access problems may distort decisions about participation in conventional clinical trials, as well as in expanded access protocols. The first involves access to health care in general (see Chapter 7). The second involves access to specific drugs.

Primary Care

The AIDS epidemic has had a disproportionate impact on the urban poor in the United States. Socioeconomic factors associated with high rates of intravenous drug abuse, such as poverty, unemployment, and inadequate education, are also associated with higher rates of HIV infection, especially in the major population centers of the Northeast. Repeated studies have shown that access to primary medical care is inadequate for the impoverished men, women, and children who are most likely to become infected with HIV. Contributing to access difficulties is the fact that the proportion of physicians practicing primary care specialties has dropped precipitously in this country over the past two decades. The number of physicians who are willing to provide primary care for Medicaid patients with HIV infection is extremely small.

One dilemma created by this situation is that patients may have to enter drug trials to obtain basic health care. All of the efforts by institutional review boards and others to ensure that participation in randomized clinical trials is voluntary may mean very little if the patient has no alternative form of care. Similarly, the patient's right to withdraw from a trial at any point is jeopardized if dropping out means losing touch with essential health care providers.

Parallel track protocols are unlikely to ease this situation because the primary care provider is the fundamental link between the patient and the drug sponsor. A patient cannot participate in a parallel track protocol unless his or her primary care physician certifies that the patient meets the requirements of the protocol and that all efforts have been made to use standard therapies. The physician also must agree to participate fully in patient education and to monitor the patient closely for adverse effects of the investigational drug.

Difficult Choices

Patients who are fortunate enough to have a primary care physician have an advocate in the search for an appropriate experimental therapy. Sometimes, however, a physician will learn that a patient is not eligible to receive a desired drug because he or she does not meet the entry criteria for relevant protocols. A San Francisco physician who encountered this situation recently polled his colleagues about how they would handle it. A surprisingly large number replied that they would ignore the entry criteria and, if necessary, falsify laboratory data rather than deny the patient access to a potentially beneficial drug.

Discussions about misrepresentation in clinical trials have focused mainly on patients who knowingly take drugs that are not authorized by a study protocol or who surreptitiously have their drugs analyzed to determine whether they have received the investigational drug or a placebo in a blinded study. The informal poll described above indicates that the problem could go much deeper. Open-label studies, such as the parallel track protocol, are especially vulnerable to misrepresentation because regulators and sponsors keep reporting requirements to a minimum.

COMPETING RIGHTS

Every time a patient or physician misrepresents a patient's clinical status to enroll the patient in a drug trial, the quality of data collected in that trial diminishes. For example, a study protocol might be designed to assess whether patients who have failed to improve on standard therapies benefit from a new investigational drug. If a patient gained entry to such a study without trying standard therapies, information related to that patient would distort conclusions drawn from the entire trial. Improvement in the patient's condition would be regarded as evidence that the drug had the potential to help a certain group of patients—those who had failed to respond to other measures—when in fact the evidence did not pertain to that group at all.

If many patients and physicians choose to follow this course, future patients will not have accurate information on which to base their own choices about treatment alternatives. The tension between the needs and rights of today's patients and the needs and rights of future patients is an unfortunate corollary of the drug evaluation process. The only way to obtain accurate information about the risks and benefits of an unknown agent is to introduce it through a series of careful, methodical clinical trials. Understandably, however, today's patients often view immediate access to a potentially beneficial drug as a higher priority than the gathering of information for future patient populations. (Sometimes, however, participants in trials are also direct beneficiaries of the results. For example, when the recent trial of AZT in patients with asymptomatic HIV infection was terminated, more than 90 percent of the participants had not yet developed AIDS and were immediately offered AZT.)

Organized expanded access may help resolve this conflict, but only if parallel track protocols do not interfere with enrollment in conventional clinical trials. Patient advocates suggest that one way to increase patient accrual in conventional trials and to decrease the risk of misrepresentation is to include patients, their advocates, and their primary care physicians in the planning of each protocol. Patient representatives can provide important insights into the factors that make a particular trial more or less appealing to the target population.

INSTITUTIONAL REVIEW BOARDS

Expanded access reflects some underlying changes in the philosophy of drug regulation, and these changes will be mirrored in the functioning of institutional review boards, the local organizations charged with protecting the rights of individuals who participate in clinical trials. These changes are subtle and do not call for eliminating the traditional concerns of IRBs; they may, however, challenge IRBs to modify and revise some commonly held principles.

First, there has been a shift in emphasis from nonmaleficence to beneficence; that is, from preventing harm by protecting patients from risk to actively promoting patients' welfare by providing them earlier and broader access to experimental drugs.

Second, a different aspect of patient autonomy is receiving more emphasis. IRBs have always been concerned with patients' rights—to be free from subtle or overt coercion in making decisions about whether or not to participate in a research protocol, to have full information to make informed choices, and to take the risks associated with participation in protocols, as long as those risks are understood. Recently IRBs have had to recognize that many patients are more concerned with their right to take serious risks than with their right to be free from coercion.

Finally, IRBs will have to adjust their perspective on the selection of subjects for participation in trials. Traditionally, IRBs have acted to protect individuals and groups from being included in trials simply because they were easily accessible—for example, prisoners—or because they were vulnerable—for instance, drug users or pregnant women. Today, when patients believe that participation in clinical trials offers substantial promise of benefit, these restrictions may be viewed as discriminatory rather than as protection from harm.

NEW ATTITUDES

The effect of the AIDS epidemic on drug regulators has not received a great deal of attention, but some observers suggest that calls for expedited development and early expanded access could have a major impact on the way regulators view their own responsibilities. For decades, regulators and drug sponsors have had an almost adversarial relationship. Sponsors produced and organized huge amounts of data and presented it to the FDA for evaluation. The FDA played the devil's advocate, often focusing more on the potential for adverse effects than on the potential benefits of a candidate drug. Regulators were rewarded for refusing marketing privileges to a drug or device that later turned out to be harmful; there were no comparable rewards for making a beneficial drug available quickly.

Advocates for patients with many different diseases have complained that the traditional system placed too much emphasis on caution. But some scientists and legislators worry that new procedures could err in the other direction. If FDA officials become deeply involved in the design of drug protocols, will they still be objective when the time comes to evaluate the data generated by those protocols? If a protocol does not exactly answer the questions that must be addressed to assess safety and efficacy, will the regulator who helped shape the protocol be willing to turn to sponsors and suggest starting over?

Identifying promising drugs and getting them to the marketplace as quickly as possible are extremely worthwhile goals, but everyone should be aware of the potential costs as well as the potential benefits. For example, the new emphasis on expedited development greatly increases the demands on postmarketing testing and surveillance systems. Drugs could be approved for marketing even if some questions remained about the most effective ways to use them. Physicians who treat patients with drugs approved through expedited review must understand the importance of responding quickly to all requests for information and of relaying all questions and concerns to drug sponsors as they arise.

3

EVALUATION OF EXPANDED ACCESS PROGRAMS

Scientists have only begun to formulate the questions that will need to be addressed to determine whether the benefits of very early access to AIDS drugs exceed the risks. Experience with the treatment IND program and with other forms of early access may help guide the evaluation process.

TREATMENT INVESTIGATIONAL NEW DRUGS

The treatment IND regulations issued by the FDA in May 1987 were greeted with great enthusiasm by persons with AIDS and their advocates. They viewed the regulations as a dramatic shift in FDA policies that would allow hundreds or thousands of patients to gain access to investigational drugs. Three years later, however, many AIDS activists consider the program a failure. Although six treatment INDs for AIDS-related drugs have been approved, the activists say that the treatment IND accomplishes too little, too late.

The underlying problem, described in Chapter 1, is that patients and FDA officials had very different expectations about what the treatment IND would accomplish. FDA officials regarded the rules as an opportunity to make drugs available to patients with life-threatening conditions and no treatment alternatives, but only after the acquisition of clinical evidence that a drug was relatively safe and probably effective. Early charts produced by the FDA showed that approval of a treatment IND would be most likely for drugs nearing the end of the traditional phase 2 clinical trial; or, if the condition

---

This chapter is based on the presentations of Robert Temple, Jay Lipner, Lawrence Corey, Raphael Dolin, Bernard Lo, Jerome Birnbaum, and Susan Ellenberg.

was "serious" but not life-threatening, the treatment IND might be approved during the phase 3 trial.   AIDS patients, on the other hand, expected the treatment IND to make drugs available at a very early stage of development.

Problems with the treatment IND demonstrate the importance of early and consistent communication.   Efforts to include patients, primary care physicians, and AIDS activists in the planning process might prevent similar problems from arising with the new parallel track program.

POTENTIAL RISKS

Drug regulators have indicated their willingness to begin parallel track programs concurrently with the beginning of phase 2 trials. Patients and their physicians must understand, however, that scientists may have very little information about the potential adverse effects of a drug at that time.

Consider, for example, a phase 1 trial involving 20 patients. Statisticians explain that even if no serious toxicities were observed in those 20 patients, the upper 95 percent confidence limit for the true serious toxicity rate would be 17 percent (as many as 1 in 6 patients might experience a severe toxic reaction).   Even if the phase 1 trial were expanded to 40 patients with no adverse effects, the true toxicity rate could be as high as 9 percent.

If physicians observed one serious reaction among 20 patients in a phase 1 trial, the observed rate would be 5 percent, but the true rate could be as high as 25 percent. A patient considering enrollment in a parallel track protocol might feel very differently about a 1-in-20 chance of a severe adverse reaction than about a 1-in-4 chance.

Examples from the Past

A study in the early 1970s of a potential treatment for herpes encephalitis provides a more graphic illustration of some of the problems that can arise with expanded access protocols.   Herpes encephalitis is a life-threatening infection of the brain caused by the herpes simplex virus.   In the late 1960s and early 1970s, about half a dozen case reports in the medical literature described treatment of this disease with a new drug called 5-iododeoxyuridine (IUDR). Scientists had a strong rationale for IUDR's antiviral effects and there were no treatment alternatives, so the FDA quickly approved an open-label IND. Infectious disease specialists came to regard IUDR as the treatment of choice for herpes encephalitis and administered it to more than 70 patients under the open-label IND.

After several years, however, investigators decided to take a closer look at the drug's effects. Despite the objections of some early pioneers in the field, they organized a small placebo-controlled, randomized study. (The pioneers had believed that a placebo-controlled trial would be unethical because of existing clinical evidence in favor of the drug.) The results of the placebo-controlled study were striking. Of the 12 patients who received IUDR, 9 had some evidence of serious toxicity (an estimated 3 to 5 died as a direct result of the drug's adverse effects on bone marrow). Moreover, autopsy results in 4 patients who received IUDR showed that the patients had virus in the brain at the end of therapy. This example shows that even those who are acknowledged experts in a medical field may have difficulty predicting the benefit/risk ratio for a new investigational drug.

The Target Population

Physicians enrolling patients in expanded access protocols also should understand the potential impact of demographic differences on the outcome of clinical trials. These differences are important first in interpreting risk based on phase 1 trials and later in comparing phase 2 clinical trials with corresponding parallel track protocols.

Conventional clinical trials generally have very specific requirements with regard to the health status of prospective subjects. Scientists want to be able to see the effects of an investigational drug with a minimum of interference from other drugs, from confounding diseases, or from other risk factors. In HIV infection, age and overall health status affect survival and the rate of progression of disease; nutrition, past smoking history, and past occupational status affect the frequency of disseminated opportunistic infections (especially fungal and mycobacterial infections). To control for these differences among patients, differences that could confound the findings of a study, most investigators attempt to make their study populations as homogeneous as possible. In contrast, parallel track protocols enable thousands of patients with diverse backgrounds and medical histories to get access to drugs after minimal testing in a highly selected subgroup. The incidence of adverse effects in patients weakened by repeated battles with *Pneumocystis carinii* and other microorganisms, or by the effects of intravenous drug abuse, could be very different from that observed in the relatively healthier population characteristic of the phase 2 trial.

The recent controversy over ddI illustrates some of the problems that can arise when people try to make direct comparisons between expanded access programs and conventional phase 2 trials. In March 1990, a spokesman for Bristol-Myers Squibb told a reporter from the *New York Times* that the death rate among patients in the parallel track protocol for ddI was 10 times higher than the death rate among patients enrolled in phase 2 trials of the drug. Of the almost 8,000 patients enrolled in the expanded access program, 290 had died; in contrast, only 2 of 700 patients in the phase 2 trials had died.

These figures were used to illustrate the dangers of expanded access, and physicians received hundreds of telephone calls from worried patients. Yet initial reviews of the data indicated that most or even all of the disparity might be due to the fact that patients in the expanded access program were sicker to begin with than patients in the clinical trials. With the exception of six deaths from pancreatitis (five in the expanded access program and one in the phase 2 trial), the deaths seemed to result from natural progression of the disease. (However, complete data from both protocols have not yet been published.)

The expanded access protocols for ddI were designed for patients who could not meet eligibility requirements for participation in the clinical trials. The majority have been intolerant of or unresponsive to zidovudine (AZT). Many cannot participate in the conventional trials because they are taking medications such as gancyclovir to fight severe opportunistic infections. Others are too sick to undertake the time and travel commitments necessary for participation in a traditional drug trial. All of these characteristics are indicative of progressive disease.

Safety Data

The proposed policy statement on the parallel track developed within the Public Health Service indicates that all physicians participating in a parallel track protocol should be required to report safety data (the collection of efficacy data depends on the specific protocol; see Chapter 4). Some observers have suggested that this requirement is too stringent—that mandatory reporting should not be part of a program designed primarily to increase access to therapy for desperately ill patients with no treatment alternatives. They worry that even minimal reporting requirements will discourage participation by physicians and by drug sponsors (who assume financial responsibility for data collection).

Although these concerns are genuine, they represent a failure to appreciate the risks involved in widespread use of minimally tested agents. Failure to request reports of serious events in the parallel track could delay recognition of severe side effects for months or even years, increasing potential risks for patients enrolled in both research and open protocols.

IMPACT ON CONVENTIONAL RANDOMIZED TRIALS

In addition to worries about safety, critics of the parallel track have expressed great concern about its effects on enrollment in traditional clinical trials. Randomized, controlled trials provide definitive information about the relative risks and benefits of new therapies. Sponsors must have such information to seek approval for marketing from the FDA. Marketing, in turn, is the most efficient way to make a drug available to large numbers of people.

The critics are concerned that patients will enter the parallel track to avoid the uncertainty of a randomized trial. They refer to news articles about individuals who have sought outside help to identify drugs they receive in blinded studies as evidence that patients will not participate in a traditional clinical trial if other options are available. Supporters of the parallel track believe that current screening mechanisms are sufficient to separate people who are eligible for clinical trials from those who are eligible for the parallel track. They suggest that improved patient education and better trial design (see Chapter 4) will ensure patient accrual in the randomized trials and, at the same time, allow patients who are ineligible for clinical trials to receive experimental drugs through expanded access programs.

The experience with ddI highlights some early mistakes. Bristol-Myers Squibb received the exclusive license for ddI from the National Cancer Institute (NCI) in mid-1988. During the late summer and early fall of 1988, the NCI and Bristol-Myers Squibb sponsored four separate phase 1 trials of the drug. These trials produced a reasonable expectation that ddI was efficacious against HIV and that it was safe enough to allow expansion of a clinical program.

The company worked with the NCI, the National Institute of Allergy and Infectious Diseases (NIAID), and the FDA to develop appropriate phase 2/3 trials. At the FDA's request, the company submitted a proposal for a treatment IND; it also worked closely with AIDS patients and their representatives to develop a prototype parallel track protocol.   The FDA approved the phase 2/3 trials and the expanded access protocols on September 28, 1989.   The first patient was placed on the expanded access protocol on October 12. The drug was shipped to the first phase 2 investigators on October 11, but actual enrollment of patients did not begin until October 20.

Many observers believe that the lag time between the start-up of the parallel track and the beginning of the phase 2/3 trials may have distorted the enrollment process.   Patients who were eligible for the clinical trials entered the parallel track because ddI was not available any other way (excessive expectations for ddI created by the news media may have been partly responsible for this problem).   An important lesson for future parallel track programs has been learned, that is, to ensure that enrollment in clinical trials precedes or coincides with the release of drugs through the parallel track protocol.

To this day, much controversy remains over the question of whether or not the availability of ddI through the parallel track has adversely effected accrual to the three clinical trials of ddI (protocol 116, a comparison of AZT versus ddI in recently diagnosed AIDS and ARC patients; protocol 117, a comparison of AZT versus ddI in patients who have been on AZT for longer than 12 months; and protocol 118, a dose-escalating trial of ddI in AIDS-intolerant persons).   Views range from the belief that the expanded access program had very little effect on accrual to the trials, to the belief that the expanded access program has had a disastrous effect.   As of January 1991, there were more than 14,000 patients receiving ddI through expanded access programs and approximately 1,600 patients participating in the trials, which are about 75 percent filled.   Most scientists associated with the trials seem to feel that some eligible patients must have been diverted from the trials by expanded access. They assert that, although the rates of accrual to the ACTG trials of ddI have been similar to rates for trials of other AIDS drugs, without the competing availability of ddI through expanded access these trials would have recruited patients much more quickly.

THE PARALLEL TRACK EXPERIMENT

Although expanded access has been part of the drug evaluation system for many years, the formal parallel track approach is new. The proposal for the approach states that the entire parallel track program for AIDS drugs should be regarded as a pilot test.   Many investigators would like to see mechanisms built into the program to answer questions about differential toxicity rates and about the impact of the parallel track on clinical trials. The Public Health Service plans to organize a working group to assess the parallel track concept, but their task will be quite difficult unless data collection and certain evaluation strategies are incorporated into parallel track protocols from the beginning.

The extent of data collection efforts to be included in the parallel track is a complex issue. Ideally, basic demographic data and some clinical indicators of efficacy and toxicity should be collected in a format similar to that used for conventional clinical trials. It may be difficult, however, to convey state-of-the-art staging information to the broad spectrum of physicians who wish to enroll patients in the parallel track. Given that the primary goal of the parallel track is to make drugs accessible to desperately ill patients, sponsors must strive to obtain basic information without discouraging physician participation.

One option may be to arrange for a subset of patients in the parallel track to be followed by persons or institutions who are also involved in conventional trials of a candidate drug. Academic medical centers, CPCRA groups (members of the Community Programs for Clinical Research on AIDS), and other community-based research groups could be recruited for such a task. Data collection on these patients would be more comprehensive than that required for other parallel track participants but not as extensive as that specified for the ACTG trials. This strategy would permit comparisons of outcome and toxicity on two different levels: (1) between subjects enrolled in clinical trials and the subgroup of parallel track participants followed in a fairly rigorous fashion and (2) between the subgroup and the larger population of parallel track patients. The results could give government scientists, drug sponsors, and HIV-infected patients and their physicians a foundation for evaluating the parallel track program.

4

CREATIVITY IN CLINICAL TRIALS

Each month physicians participating in the expanded access protocols for ddI submit status reports on their patients to the drug sponsor and, in return, receive new supplies of the drug. The clinical and laboratory data enable the sponsor and government scientists to monitor the course of the protocols—especially with regard to safety concerns as described in Chapter 3. But the availability of these data also raises questions about the role of expanded access in the drug evaluation process. Can the information gathered through expanded access be used to speed or enhance the evaluation of AIDS drugs?

The answer to this question depends on a host of medical, scientific, and financial issues. Chapters 5 and 6 examine the costs of the parallel track approach for drug sponsors, patients, and third-party payers. This chapter explores the drive for innovation in clinical trials and the possibility of including expanded access protocols as part of the broad spectrum of drug evaluation mechanisms.

THE CHANGING ENVIRONMENT

Since the beginning of the AIDS epidemic, persons infected with HIV and their advocates have complained about the conservative nature of the drug development and evaluation process. Many have viewed the strict entry criteria for these clinical trials as an unreasonable barrier to participation. The problem grows worse as greater numbers of patients reach the advanced stages of HIV

This chapter is based on the presentations of Lincoln Moses, Lawrence Corey, Melanie Thompson, Marvin Zelen, Floyd J. Fowler, Susan Ellenberg, and Ellen Cooper.

infection. Each new opportunistic infection decreases the chances that a patient will qualify for entry into a desired clinical trial. One physician reports screening 80 to 100 patients to find 5 who qualified for any of the formal clinical trials of ddI. Another physician screened 275 patients to enroll 35 in the ddI trials. The extensive screening procedures slow patient accrual and lengthen the time required for completion of clinical trials. Moreover, when patients are excluded from a trial investigators lose the opportunity to learn anything from those patients, including information about drug-drug or drug-disease interactions, and how sicker patients respond to the drugs under study.

Some scientists also question the relevance of clinical trials conducted with a highly selected subgroup of the population. As HIV-infected patients live longer, their clinical histories become more diverse; they have different opportunistic infections and receive different combinations of drugs. Clinical trials that ignore these differences—that focus exclusively on a homogeneous group of patients—may not provide an accurate perspective on the drug's performance in the real world.

Most government scientists, academics, and patient representatives agree that there are many opportunities for greater creativity in the clinical trials process. Scientists are exploring new ways to modify the standard three-phase approach to drug evaluation—to improve efficiency without undermining the reliability of results. Other proposals include establishing preference trials, devising large-scale trials with broad eligibility requirements and limited data collection (similar to the International Studies of Infarct Survival in Europe), and gathering data through the parallel track.

CONVENTIONAL TRIALS

Decades of experience indicate that conventional randomized controlled clinical trials (RCT) are the most reliable and informative way to obtain information about the safety and efficacy of an investigational drug. The IUDR story in Chapter 3 is just one example of a situation in which randomized study of a small group of patients revealed that a highly regarded treatment was not accomplishing its goal. The Cardiac Arrhythmia Suppression Trial, or CAST, provides another relevant case history.

The CAST effort involved two drugs, encainide and flecainide, both known to suppress irregular heartbeats in patients with heart disease. Many physicians believed that these drugs should be administered widely to patients who had suffered a heart attack (because deaths following a heart attack often result from irregular heart rhythms) and that it would be unethical to conduct a placebo-controlled trial in which some patients would not receive the drugs. A randomized trial was begun, however, and the results were startling. The trial demonstrated that the drugs did, indeed, reduce irregular heartbeats compared with placebo, but they also increased mortality among patients who had symptomatic but not life-threatening rhythm abnormalities.

The strength of RCTs lies in the fact that they are structured to eliminate as many extraneous differences as possible between the groups being compared. This can be accomplished by applying very carefully devised inclusion and exclusion criteria, carefully following a protocol, and, of course, assigning patients randomly to treatment arms. These procedures are especially important in HIV infection, which has an erratic clinical course and many different patterns of illness.

The challenge for AIDS investigators is to retain the advantages of traditional clinical trials and at the same time reduce entry restrictions. The AIDS Clinical Trials Group has established a Protocol Evaluation Subcommittee to explore ways to make trials more efficient and flexible. The Statistical Working Group of the ACTG is also working to broaden entry criteria for clinical trials and to speed their progress. Scientists writing new protocols have been encouraged to reduce requirements for laboratory tests and to shorten reporting forms.

But there are limits to these approaches. Some research questions require a high level of technological expertise. On the other hand, the academic medical centers that possess this expertise may not have the facilities to provide care for the full spectrum of HIV-infected patients. (Chapter 7 explores the limitations of some traditional clinical trial sites in providing care for women and people of color.) The establishment of the Community Programs for Clinical Research on AIDS (CPCRA), described in Chapter 1, is based on the concept that HIV infection raises many different types of research questions. Some are best answered within the confines of a traditional clinical trial; others are more appropriate for large, simple randomized trials in which the bulk of the patient population is treated in the community. "Low-technology" randomized trials, combined with expanded access programs, offer an opportunity to learn something from all segments of the population infected with HIV.

PREFERENCE TRIALS

Before addressing the positive features of the large, low-technology trial, it is important to examine the pros and cons of one other experimental design, the preference trial.   The preference trial is based on the concept that when treatments are tested only on select subsets of patients and a treatment effect is observed, doubt remains about how the treatment will work for most patients under less controlled circumstances.   Therefore, proponents of preference trials argue that studies of broad ranges of patients under varying conditions are necessary to discover how well treatments really work.

Patients may also have very different "utilities" with regard to the risks and benefits of experimental therapies.   For example, an HIV-infected patient may feel that the reduced energy level associated with one investigational drug is preferable to the nausea and vomiting associated with another.   Alternatively, on a more serious plane, patients may feel that the risk of a very severe adverse reaction in the present is worth the potential benefits of a decade or more of disease-free survival.   Supporters of preference trials believe that ethical research should take account of patients' values, a factor that randomized drug trials generally fail to consider.

These supporters propose trials in which all patients who might benefit from an experimental therapy are given an opportunity to choose between the new therapy and other treatment options.   The investigator's role would be to provide patients with as much information as possible about the potential risks and benefits of each option, and then to collect data about the patient's health status and quality of life as the trial progresses.   The underlying assumption is that individual values would lead patients with almost identical characteristics at the beginning of a trial to choose different treatment options.   At the end of the study, comparisons of the outcomes associated with each choice would enable scientists to estimate the relative safety and efficacy of the investigational drug.

Supporters of such trials say they have many potential advantages: (1) patients would be more likely to comply with treatment regimens that they have selected themselves; (2) patient accrual would be rapid because no patients would be turned away; (3) the subject population could reflect the broad spectrum of HIV-infected patients; and (4) the process of informing patients about potential risks and benefits would mirror events in the "real world" of clinical practice.

Critics argue that previous experience in drug investigation indicates that nonrandomized trials do not give reliable results. Too many factors can influence drug choice and clinical outcome.   For example, rapid shifts in the popularity of certain underground drug therapies among HIV-infected persons demonstrate the power of a social network in influencing patient decision making. In addition, when patients choose their own treatment options, there may be important differences among the treatment groups that influence outcome. Even very sophisticated statistical techniques cannot control for all such effects; experience indicates, in fact, that many important factors are unknown or unquantifiable.

Scientists opposed to preference trials say it would be deceptive and unethical to tell patients in a nonrandomized study that they are contributing to advances in drug therapy because the data collected in such trials do not provide definitive answers to basic questions about drug efficacy. But scientists who are currently experimenting with preference trials answer that blind insistence on randomized controlled trials as the only appropriate method for evaluating drugs has limited our ability to discover the true value of most of the treatments available today—because such trials are costly, difficult to complete, and, when completed, apply only to the particular subset of patients who met eligibility criteria. They believe that there are "good" and "bad" studies of all kinds and that alternatives to RCTs must be judged by how well they answer important questions and by the quality of their execution.

LARGE, SIMPLE RANDOMIZED TRIALS

Some of the positive features of the preference trial, such as broad patient participation, could also be achieved through large-scale, "low-technology" randomized trials similar to those developed in Europe to study cardiovascular diseases. These trials have involved endpoints that are easy to measure (such as survival or stroke) and limited data collection (the minimum possible to achieve satisfactory results). For example, in the International Studies of Infarct Survival (ISIS), tens of thousands of patients in many different health care settings were randomly assigned to groups to explore ways to increase survival after heart attacks. The second ISIS trial, ISIS-2, demonstrated that streptokinase and aspirin were both highly effective (compared with placebo) in reducing cardiovascular mortality after an acute myocardial infarction, and that the two agents together were significantly better than either agent alone. These effects were recognized despite the fact that patients had a wide range of background treatments (beta blockers, nitrates, and calcium channel blockers) and prognostic variables. The large size of the study ensured comparability of the patient groups.

Most of the European trials have involved drugs with known toxicities administered on a one-time basis (so compliance was not an issue), but some scientists believe that the format could be adapted to study HIV-related disorders. Large-scale trials among AIDS patients with broad eligibility requirements and streamlined data collection might be appropriate for answering questions about the optimal dosage (quantity and schedule) of an antiviral drug, drug combinations, drug interactions (especially with regard to prophylactic agents and treatments for opportunistic infections), and drug resistance.

With careful planning that emphasizes a factorial design,[1] virtually any HIV-infected patient who was willing to consent to randomization and who had access to a skilled primary care physician could be included in a trial of some kind. The idea would be to have an available trial for every AIDS patient. Data collection would focus primarily on such clinical endpoints as opportunistic infections, fevers, intractable diarrhea, HIV wasting syndrome, changes in stage of disease, important adverse reactions, and survival.

Registration could take place by telephone. A physician would call a central registration number and provide some initial data on the patient's medical history. The registrar would assign the patient to a protocol and, within 24 hours, send out patient consent forms, details of the protocol, drugs, and reporting forms.

Physician Participation

Large-scale AIDS trials would require the cooperation of many different segments of the health care community. Designated members of CPCRA and other community-based research groups would be logical sources of health care providers for these trials, but the ultimate goal would be to include independent physicians and their nursing and laboratory support staffs. One scientist suggests creating a roster of community physicians who have demonstrated their interest in the research process by attending special AIDS workshops or seminars. Workshop topics might include available protocols, patient

---

[1] A factorial experiment is one in which several factors are evaluated at the same time. For example, the effects of a drug may be evaluated by simultaneously varying doses and schedules; this is an example of a two-factor experiment. Factorial designs promote efficiency by addressing multiple questions simultaneously, including questions of drug-drug interactions.

consent, the collection of a core data set, staging, and ways to increase patient compliance.

For maximum efficiency, the link between specialists and primary care physicians could be maintained through a specialized computer network. The capability exists to develop extensive computer networks consisting of educational programs, bulletin boards with up-to-date information about ongoing trials (including special alerts about unexpected side effects), and electronic mail for direct access to medical consultants, nursing consultants, and data collection specialists.

Quality Control

One of the biggest challenges for the designers of large-scale AIDS trials would be to develop mechanisms for monitoring the quality of data. In addition to the usual data management strategies, some observers have suggested establishing auditing teams to visit participating physicians at random (primarily to compare patient records with information submitted to data collection centers).

DATA FROM THE PARALLEL TRACK

It is difficult to predict the ultimate importance of data collected through the parallel track and treatment INDs. Rapid implementation of large-scale randomized studies could greatly reduce the need for programs designed solely to increase access because most patients who could not qualify for current clinical trials would be eligible for trials with broadened eligibility requirements.

Efficacy Data

Whatever their size, parallel track programs are unlikely to provide substantial information about the efficacy of drug candidates. The value of data on efficacy depends on the existence of an adequate comparison or control group. The parallel track, as it is defined in the proposed PHS policy statement, does not make provisions for control groups of any kind. Although some researchers believe that important information on efficacy could be obtained using historical controls, many others feel that this method is flawed because of the dramatic changes in the treatment and prophylaxis of HIV-related disorders, in the proportions of patients from different risk groups, and in disease manifestations within risk behavior groups.

Safety Data and Related Information

The situation is quite different with regard to safety data. If early parallel track and treatment IND programs remain the only alternatives to conventional clinical trials, they could play a vital role in the identification of important adverse reactions. Some believe that they also could provide some information about "real-world" drug interactions and drug resistance.

The value of data from an individual parallel track protocol would depend on the provisions made for data collection and for monitoring data quality. There are two basic types of data collection: event driven and regular reporting (according to a predetermined schedule). In event-driven reporting, physicians fill out reports only when they observe an outcome of interest, such as an unexpected adverse event. Event-driven reporting places the least possible burden on the practicing physician (because most patients proceed through treatment without experiencing a reportable event); however, the method does not provide any basis for determining the accuracy of estimated event rates. Lack of reports could mean either that no reportable events occurred or that physicians failed to comply with reporting procedures. Requiring physicians to make regular reports substantially reduces the problem of underreporting (although it does not eliminate it entirely). Regular reporting may be crucial for situations in which thousands of patients receive very early access to an experimental agent.

The quantity of data required would depend on the drug candidate. Expanded access programs involving drugs in the final stages of the evaluation process (such as the former treatment IND for AZT), or drugs that had been tested in other contexts, might require less data from participating physicians. Reporting requirements would be more stringent for drugs that did not have an established safety record.

Monitoring the quality of data from the parallel track as a whole could be very difficult, even with regard to reporting of adverse events. A possible strategy might be to use selected subgroups of parallel track participants (such as those described in Chapter 3) to make comparisons between safety data from the parallel track and safety data from corresponding clinical trials.

Expectations

Government scientists and others caution against unrealistic expectations about the types of questions that could be answered through the parallel track. Some have expressed concern that excitement over nonrandomized expanded access protocols could detract from efforts to revitalize and improve randomized clinical trials. For example, the "safety valve" represented by the parallel track might relieve pressure to modify exclusion criteria or to take other actions that would make conventional trials more effective.

Widespread distribution of a drug through early expanded access programs also could lead to inordinate pressures to approve drugs for marketing before scientists have gathered adequate clinical evidence of safety and efficacy. The simple presence of a drug in the patient population could lead to a presumption of effectiveness that might be very hard to dispel. Such pressures might result in approval of a drug for a tightly defined patient group, such as patients intolerant to or failing standard therapies. Experience indicates, however, that once a drug is in the marketplace some physicians will use it in ways that are not supported by any data in the hope that it will have greater benefits (with acceptable toxicity) than standard treatments.

5

DRUG INNOVATION AND THE PHARMACEUTICAL INDUSTRY

Treatment INDs for ddI and several non-AIDS drugs demonstrate that some large pharmaceutical companies have the resources to distribute investigational drugs to thousands of patients across the country, but new expanded access programs could test the limits of these resources. Industry spokespersons have expressed concern that expectations created by parallel track and other expanded access programs could begin to affect the way in which companies make decisions about product development. In the most troublesome scenario, companies would weigh expenses associated with expanded access against future profits and decide that AIDS drugs simply did not represent a good investment. As a result, some potentially successful AIDS therapies would not be developed.

The effects of adverse incentives created by expanded access would be evident first in smaller companies, particularly the fledgling biotechnology firms. These companies have the expertise to make major strides in the new field of rational drug design, but they may not have the resources to sustain premarket drug distribution.

Ultimately, the impact of expanded access on drug innovation in AIDS will depend on three issues: (1) the possibility that expanded access programs might delay commercialization of target drugs or of other drug candidates, either by raising safety concerns or by creating an environment in which controlled trials cannot be carried out; (2) the extent to which expanded access programs increase the direct costs of drug development; and (3) the perception of risk associated with expanded access, particularly with regard to product liability.

This chapter is based on the presentations of Patrick Gage, Stephen Sherwin, Jerome Birnbaum, Paul De Stefano, Lawrence Corey, and James Bigo.

Treatment IND regulations stipulate that under some circumstances a manufacturer may charge for an experimental drug, but solely to recover costs. The proposed policy statement for the parallel track contains a brief reference to the treatment IND ruling but does not explore further the issue of drug costs. The policy of the Pharmaceutical Manufacturers Association is that the drug sponsor should bear the cost of any drug administered before market approval—in clinical trials or through expanded access protocols. So far, only one sponsor of an AIDS drug has sought payment under existing IND regulations.

TIME TO COMMERCIALIZATION

Previous chapters have emphasized the importance of making sure that expanded access programs do not delay FDA approval of effective drugs by slowing patient accrual in randomized clinical trials. After all, access to a drug is greatest when the drug is on the pharmacist's shelf. Pharmaceutical manufacturers also are concerned about the possible loss of income. In most cases, manufacturers do not begin to make a return on their investment in a drug until the FDA has reviewed all safety and efficacy data and approved the drug for marketing. Thus, the perception that a government agency might request an expanded access protocol for a drug and that such a protocol could delay the time to commercialization might lead a manufacturer to forgo development of that drug.

A spokesman for Bristol-Myers Squibb notes that time and energy invested in the expanded access protocols for ddI have caused delays in market approval for two other drugs, both antibiotics in the late stages of clinical development. He says that the opportunity cost associated with these delays—the nonrecoverable loss of future sales resulting from reductions in useful patent life—might emerge as the largest single cost factor of the expanded access effort.

DIRECT COSTS OF EXPANDED ACCESS

A brief recounting of Bristol-Myers Squibb's experience with ddI demonstrates the full range of expenses associated with an effective expanded access program. At the request of the FDA, the company submitted a treatment IND application for ddI on August 15, 1989.

Manpower Needs

A company spokesperson recalled the coordination required to provide physicians and potential recipients of ddI with necessary information, to evaluate patient eligibility, and to manage the vast quantities of data generated by the expanded access program.

In July of 1989 we had decided to locate our ddI (trade named Videx) product information center for expanded access at our U.S. Pharmaceutical Division at Evansville, Indiana. The objective was to be operational by early September.

We immediately assembled a project team. Our Medical Department gathered and organized the information necessary to manage the expanded access project and worked with our Research Division and the FDA to develop and process the ddI protocols.

Our Operations Group had the task of finding a building to house the information center and equipping it. Customer service representatives and other personnel were hired and trained. The staff at MIS [Management Information Systems] designed the computer system needed to handle physician and patient data. Our Marketing Group coordinated the information and communications elements. The Clinical Supply Group in the Research Division made preparations for the actual distribution of the drug.

Just 35 days after the project started, the Videx Information Center was a reality. To date, our ddI hotline has handled over 30,000 calls from physicians and patients. We have sent out 3,566 ddI binders and enrolled 7,545 patients [as of March 11, 1990].

The system works as follows: The physician calls our AIDS hotline. A data package and enrollment forms are sent the same day. The physician returns the completed forms, and the Center's medical staff evaluates the forms for patient eligibility. Within 72 hours of receiving the application, a month's supply of ddI is shipped or the physician is advised of patient ineligibility. Follow-up information from day 15 is provided to Bristol-Myers Squibb by day 30. Drug supplies for the second month are shipped upon receipt of this information.

In short, Bristol-Myers Squibb renovated a building, established warehouse space and shipping facilities, installed a comprehensive communications system, developed a computer system for data storage and retrieval, and set up hard-copy record storage. In addition, they produced a four-part ddI registration kit that included study protocols, patient eligibility information, the necessary registration documents, and the ddI investigator's brochure.

Additional manpower costs (primarily medical and regulatory affairs personnel) have been devoted to monitoring the expanded access program. For example, the company has established a system of onsite protocol audits to gauge reporting of adverse effects. Professional staff also make a concerted effort to keep clinical investigators in the ACTG, government scientists, and AIDS patients and their representatives informed about any new developments in the various clinical trials and expanded access protocols.

Drug Costs

The drug itself is a major cost factor. Early in development, the unit cost of a drug is high because the manufacturer has not had an opportunity to optimize strategies for formulation, packaging, labeling, quality control, and shipping. Also, the volume of production may be relatively low, so the manufacturer cannot take advantage of economies of scale.

Drug costs in expanded access programs for AIDS drugs may be particularly high because thousands of patients require long-term treatment. The need to formulate drugs in different dosage strengths also adds to the cost. Bristol-Myers Squibb has produced ddI in three different dosages to accommodate patients of different weights.

The Small Manufacturer

Large pharmaceutical companies, such as Bristol-Myers Squibb and Burroughs Wellcome (the manufacturer of AZT), appear to have the manpower and financial resources to manage expanded access protocols, at least in the short term; this may not be true for smaller firms. A spokesman for Genentech (the largest of the new biotechnology companies) noted that most small companies would have difficulty marshaling the manpower required to provide administrative support for the parallel track.

Companies like Genentech often have to seek outside funding (for example, R&D [research and development] limited partnerships) to finance basic clinical trials and to support the documentation tasks required for FDA approval. The demand created by expanded access protocols would be a further drain on resources. Biotechnology companies would have to begin the difficult process of scaling up production of recombinant proteins long before they had any chance of generating revenues. In some cases, they might have difficulty producing sufficient quantities of a drug for both randomized trials and expanded access.

These concerns have led one biotechnology executive to suggest a cost-recovery program in which companies would be permitted to charge for expanded access drugs. The arrangement would be similar to that described in the treatment IND and medical device regulations. This kind of program, however, would be effective only if patients had some mechanism to pay for the drugs, either through government sponsorship or through expansion of private health care coverage (see Chapter 6).

Patient advocates and some scientists involved in the drug development process are uncomfortable with this proposal. They say that most administrative costs associated with expanded access could be recaptured when a candidate drug receives market approval; for example, physician and patient education programs and drug distribution mechanisms in the parallel track could become the core of the commercial marketing program.

Critics also express concern about the potential of expanded access to distort the clinical trials process. If manufacturers could recoup costs prior to market approval, wide distribution under a treatment IND or parallel track might become a goal in itself. Companies might have less incentive to complete randomized trials to collect definitive evidence about the safety and efficacy of a drug.

For now, the latter concern is primarily theoretical. The basic cost issues, however, represent a practical barrier that may have to be addressed more fully by the architects of the expanded access concept.

PRODUCT LIABILITY

Smaller companies also are exceedingly sensitive to the potential for expensive legal actions. In the past, almost all drug-related product liability cases have involved agents already on the market. The expectation has been that subjects in clinical trials would not bring suit against drug manufacturers because the subjects had decided to participate in a research protocol knowing that there were risks involved in taking experimental drugs. Recently, however, suits brought against some manufacturers for adverse reactions sustained during drug trials have created an air of uncertainty for manufacturers. The law is unsettled with regard to liability for investigational drugs, and this uncertainty creates a perception of liability that may deter innovation.

Pharmaceutical manufacturers incorporate liability concerns into decisions about which agents to develop and bring to market. Representatives of small and medium-sized companies suggest that the push for expanded access could increase the perception of liability for some drug candidates, thereby making them less attractive to potential sponsors.

Concerns Specific to the Parallel Track

Three features of the parallel track heighten concern about product liability. The first is timing. Parallel track protocols are slated to begin very early in the drug development process—long before the sponsor has definitive information about the potential severity of adverse effects.

The second feature is the large number of participants. Administering a relatively unknown drug to 150 persons in a phase 2 trial is very different, in terms of potential lawsuits, from administering the drug to 5,000 patients in an expanded access protocol.

The third issue is the diversity of health care providers. In a traditional drug trial, the pharmaceutical manufacturer depends on skilled clinical investigators to provide the highest level of medical care. These clinical researchers have access to sophisticated technology to help them monitor patients and to recognize the onset of adverse reactions. Many physician participants in expanded access protocols will not have research experience. Also, some physicians will see only a few patients on a parallel track protocol; they might have more trouble spotting the side effects of an investigational drug than someone who has 50 patients on the same protocol.

Potential Solutions

Observers have suggested several mechanisms to diminish the impact of liability concerns on decisions related to AIDS drugs.

• In *Brown* v. *Superior Court*, the California Supreme Court recently eliminated strict liability (liability without fault) for pharmaceutical products. Instead, plaintiffs must prove actual negligence on the part of the companies. Some other states have similar tort rules, but in general, inconsistency is the rule on the issue among the states. If this doctrine could be extended to apply to investigational drugs, companies might be reassured.

• Another reform would be to implement the so-called government standards defense. Under this theory, a company that has complied with the FDA requirements for approval has a legal defense to a negligence claim. This mechanism would prevent judges or juries from second-guessing the conclusions of the regulatory agency. However, it might be difficult to extend this form of legal protection to products not yet approved by the FDA.

• Product liability decisions are made by state courts. If the federal government stepped in to standardize these rules nationally, manufacturers would consider this action a large step forward.

• A final mechanism would be to amend existing FDA regulations to make it possible for pharmaceutical manufacturers to negotiate directly with prospective subjects in clinical trials, who would then waive their right to sue. The FDA usually does not permit this type of one-on-one negotiation, but an industry lawyer suggests that it might be appropriate in the context of expanded access programs for AIDS drugs because patients and their physicians assume greater responsibility for the decision to proceed with treatment than do participants in traditional clinical trials.

6

THIRD-PARTY PAYERS

Most expanded access drugs have been provided "free of charge" to patients, but this term can be misleading. For example, Bristol-Myers Squibb has not charged patients for ddI under the treatment IND or parallel track protocols, but patients cannot participate in these protocols unless their physicians send monthly follow-up reports to the company about their health status. These reports must include the results of laboratory tests that cost between $100 and $300. Neither the company nor, in many cases, third-party payers will reimburse patients for these charges. Thus, even though the drug is free, either the patient or the health care system must absorb a substantial amount of drug-related charges.

The parallel track concept has arisen at a time of considerable turmoil in the U.S. health care system. Widespread concern over the high cost of medical care in the United States has placed great pressure on both public and private third-party payers to minimize expenditures. At the same time, government policymakers have been bombarded by studies showing a severe shortage of basic health care services for major segments of the population, particularly low-income minorities in urban centers.

This environment provides a particularly difficult setting in which to resolve questions about payment for health care services related to investigational drugs. Traditionally, third-party payers have covered services that are reasonable and necessary for the treatment of illness or injury. With respect to drugs, this has meant drugs recognized by the FDA as safe and effective—in other words, drugs that are

---

This chapter is based on the presentations of David Higbee, Susan Gleeson, Steven Peskin, Lee Mortenson, and Daniel Hoth.

considered part of standard medical practice. Most third-party contracts specifically exclude coverage of investigational drugs.

Although such policies seem straightforward, they leave considerable room for interpretation. For example, when a severely ill patient receives an investigational drug, how much of that patient's care is attributable to the investigational protocol and how much would have been required in any case? Also, how should one handle costs for a disease such as AIDS, in which the appropriate and medically required treatment for a patient may be investigational in nature? Finally, how should third-party payers assess coverage for FDA-approved drugs used in ways that are not specified on the drug's FDA-approved label?

Some patient advocates claim that worsening economic conditions in health care have caused third-party payers to become increasingly restrictive in their reimbursement policies. In certain situations, they say, a patient's decision to enter a clinical trial has led insurers to refuse reimbursement for hospitalization, physician fees, and patient care costs that would have been required even if the patient had not been involved in a research protocol. They worry that such behavior will have a negative effect on drug innovation; physicians and institutions that become wary about reimbursement policies might stop entering their patients in clinical trials.

Patient advocates also express concern about the emphasis on drug labels; they say that they have seen a growing tendency to restrict reimbursement for FDA-approved drugs to indications specified on the drug label. They suggest that this practice, and the related practice of requiring prior approval for reimbursement of unlabeled indications, interfere with the physician's ability to provide good medical care. For example, a representative of the Association of Community Cancer Centers reports that there are 12 indications for interferon specified in the *U.S. Pharmacopoeia* (USP), but only 3 are listed on the FDA label.

Third-party payers, on the other hand, say that they have responded as quickly as possible to a series of very rapid shifts in medical practice, especially with regard to new therapies. A spokeswoman for Blue Cross and Blue Shield uses recent changes in the treatment IND program to illustrate this situation. From the perspective of third-party payers, she says, the treatment IND was supposed to act as a bridge from phase 3 trials to FDA approval. Suddenly, however, the FDA approved a treatment IND for ddI, which had not even entered phase 2 trials.

Blue Cross and Blue Shield, the Health Insurance Association of America (which represents about 320 independent insurance companies in the United States), and the Health Care Financing Administration (HCFA; which administers Medicare and Medicaid) have all begun to reexamine their policies with regard to reimbursement for clinical trials and off-label uses of FDA-approved drugs.

BLUE CROSS AND BLUE SHIELD

Among Blue Cross and Blue Shield plans, 89 percent pay hospital and physician charges for patients in clinical trials when the hospitalization is medically necessary, independent of the investigational treatment. Eleven percent do not pay these standard patient care costs.

A representative of the Blue Cross and Blue Shield Association explains that each of the 74 plans nationwide makes its own decisions about coverage. Often, however, the decisions are based on recommendations made by the association's nationally recognized technology assessment programs. Recently, the association began a study of reimbursement for patient care costs, with special emphasis on clinical trials. The study will look at coverage issues that arise when one or both arms of a trial involve standard therapies. Staff members hope to develop a classification system that will help Blue Cross and Blue Shield plans assess future research protocols.

Last year, the association and plans adopted a new position on FDA labeling. In the past, reimbursement was limited to labeled indications; now, most Blue Cross and Blue Shield plans will reimburse for off-label indications if there is specific evidence of efficacy. Such evidence may come from one of the major drug compendia or from a plan's own assessment of existing research. In addition to efficacy and safety data, a plan may look for evidence that the desired drug is at least as beneficial as existing therapies. (Some patient advocates say that this new position is actually a retreat because many plans paid for off-label indication as part of standard patient care costs in the absence of an official policy.)

The Blue Cross and Blue Shield Association has a mixed record with respect to expanded access programs for investigational drugs. Last year, after considerable debate, the association advised plans that it would continue to view Group C cancer drugs as investigational, largely because plan contracts say that a drug must have final approval from the FDA to be payable. However, the plans did pay for the AIDS-related drug aerosolized pentamidine when it was distributed under a treatment IND (this may have been related to the fact that pentamidine already was approved by the FDA for intravenous administration).

The association's overall policy on HIV infection is that it should be treated just like any other disease. At the beginning of the epidemic, the central question was how to manage benefits in the absence of effective therapies. A large Blue Cross and Blue Shield task force recommended that plans adopt the case management approach, a strategy for assessing the circumstances of individual patient cases and making exceptions to standard contracts in an organized fashion.

Services that may be reimbursed under the case management approach include counseling, home care, and hospice care. Blue Shield of California has used the case management approach to supplement services provided by local community groups. Blue Cross and Blue Shield of Massachusetts is exploring the use of case management (under a cost-sharing agreement with participating teaching hospitals) to cover investigational treatments for life-threatening diseases that lack alternative remedies. A representative of Blue Cross and Blue Shield says that case management probably will remain the primary strategy for accommodating the special needs of patients with AIDS and other life-threatening diseases. She does not anticipate any specific contract changes.

Some patient advocates greet such news with concern. They believe that it is illogical to treat vast numbers of patients by exception. In addition, they fear that uncertainties about coverage and delays in reimbursement will discourage physicians from treating AIDS patients. Case management will become more difficult, they say, as more patients progress to the later stages of HIV infection.

HEALTH INSURANCE ASSOCIATION OF AMERICA

The Health Insurance Association of America (HIAA) is the largest trade association for the commercial insurance industry. The companies it represents underwrite about 85 percent of all commercial health insurance in the United States. Recently, HIAA convened a task force to make recommendations to member companies about off-label uses of approved drugs, treatment IND drugs, Group C drugs, and related issues. The recommendations encourage companies to be flexible, especially with regard to drugs for immediately life-threatening conditions.

For example, the task force suggested that member companies refer to three national compendia in assessing reimbursement for off-label uses of FDA-approved drugs. They are the *American Hospital Formulary Service Drug Information*, the *American Medical Association*

Drug Evaluations, and the *U.S. Pharmacopoeia Drug Information*. In addition, the task force recommended that insurers study the peer-reviewed literature and seek guidance directly from the research community. For immediately life-threatening conditions—patients with no other hope—the task force encouraged consideration of novel approaches that might not have received full peer review.

With regard to investigational drugs, the task force recommended that drugs for immediately life-threatening or serious conditions be considered for coverage—or at least not categorically denied—by health insurers. This includes treatment IND drugs and Group C cancer drugs. The task force also advised member companies to reimburse for costs associated with hospitalization for multidrug regimens involving a combination of approved and investigational drugs. (The experimental drugs themselves would not be covered; typically, these drugs are paid for by the pharmaceutical company or through research grants.) The task force did not recommend reimbursement for hospitalizations associated with single-drug clinical investigations. (Again, however, exceptions might be made for drugs for immediately life-threatening conditions.)

A spokesman for the task force said that the industry would welcome greater input from the FDA in evaluating the efficacy of investigational drugs. He also recommended the development of an alternative to tort remedy for fair, equitable, and expedient adjudication of disputes over drug coverage denials.

Patient advocates applaud HIAA's recognition of the three major compendia for assessing off-label uses of approved drugs and the recommendations concerning payment of hospital and patient care costs for multidrug clinical trials. They add, however, that it is too early to judge the impact of the recommendations because it is not clear whether member companies will follow them. Moreover, evidence from several studies indicates that the proportion of AIDS patients who are covered by private health insurance has declined over time. This trend probably will continue as the demographics of the epidemic continue to change. In addition, a 1988 survey by the congressional Office of Technology Assessment (OTA) found that commercial insurance companies, along with Blue Cross and Blue Shield plans and health maintenance organizations, were planning to reduce their exposure to the financial impact of AIDS. (Possible strategies included reducing sales to individuals and small group markets through tighter underwriting guidelines, expanding the use of HIV and other testing, adding AIDS-related questions to enrollment applications, and denying coverage to applicants with a history of sexually transmitted diseases.) Some commercial carriers have placed dollar limits on AIDS coverage in new policies and others have introduced waiting periods for AIDS benefits. In this environment, the positive effects of HIAA's new policies on drug coverage might be relatively limited with respect to HIV-related disorders.

HEALTH CARE FINANCING ADMINISTRATION

Three years ago, the Health Care Financing Administration of the Department of Health and Human Services estimated that 40 percent of all patients with AIDS were served under Medicaid. This figure probably has increased substantially as a result of the growing proportion of cases associated with intravenous drug abuse. In some areas, such as New York and New Jersey, the proportion of patients covered by Medicaid may be as high as 70 percent. Medicare, in contrast, covers fewer than 2 percent of AIDS patients.

Medicaid

Drug coverage under Medicaid varies tremendously among states because it is considered an optional service; the only statutory guideline is that states may not receive federal payment for drugs that have not been determined effective by the FDA. Coverage of investigational drugs and of unlabeled indications of approved drugs is usually at the discretion of the state.[1]

---

[1]In a 1989 decision, the U.S. Court of Appeals, Eighth Circuit, placed a limit on state discretion with respect to the coverage of unlabeled indications of FDA-approved drugs. The case challenged a Missouri Medicaid rule precluding certain Medicaid recipients with AIDS from receiving reimbursement for AZT. The Missouri regulations limited coverage for AZT to patients who had a history of cytologically confirmed *Pneumocystis carinii* pneumonia (PCP) or an absolute CD4 lymphocyte count of less than 200 per cubic millimeter in the peripheral blood before therapy (limitations stipulated in the FDA approval statement for the drug). The court concluded, "the fact that FDA has not approved labeling of a drug for a particular use does not necessarily bear on those uses of the drug that are established within the medical and scientific community as medically appropriate. It would be improper for the State of Missouri to interfere with a physician's judgment of medical necessity by limiting coverage of AZT based on criteria that admittedly do not reflect current medical knowledge or practice." The court found that Missouri Medicaid's approach to its coverage of the drug AZT was "unreasonable and inconsistent with the objectives of the Medicaid Act" (*Weaver* v. *Reagen*, 886 F.2d 194, 8th Cir., 1989).

State Discretion

A recent informal survey of 12 states conducted by HCFA staff members revealed that 7 (Colorado, Florida, Idaho, Massachusetts, Michigan, Texas, and Utah) did not allow any coverage of investigational drugs. The other 5 states—Illinois, New York, California, Iowa, and Virginia—allowed limited coverage on a case-by-case basis. For example, Medicaid coverage of an investigational drug in Illinois depends on three conditions: (1) the drug must be for the treatment of AIDS or an AIDS-related condition; (2) the drug must have official treatment IND status from the FDA; and (3) the recipient or program must be officially charged for the drug by the drug sponsor.

New York has a policy against payment for experimental medical care or services through Medicaid; however, the state will make an exception for an investigational drug if the FDA provides guidelines for the safe administration of the drug and if the guidelines meet the approval of the New York State Department of Health. When these criteria are met, determinations are made on a prior-approval basis for each individual. As of March 1990, the only drug approved for coverage in this fashion was aerosolized pentamidine.

In California, a patient's physician may request authorization for reimbursement for an investigational drug before treatment. Again, determination is made on a case-by-case basis.

Patient Care Costs

Such variation among the states raises the issue of fairness to beneficiaries of the different plans. The fairness issue becomes even more acute, however, in relation to patient care costs associated with investigational drugs. Recently, scientists have noticed that the probability of dying from AIDS increases in those patients who are on their second year of AZT therapy. This observation leads many to believe that the positive effects of AZT may begin to "wear off" in many AIDS patients after 12 to 18 months. For thousands of patients, the only remaining therapeutic alternative is an investigational drug.

Drug sponsors or research grants usually pay drug-related patient care costs for individuals enrolled in traditional clinical trials, but there are no similar arrangements for patients receiving drugs through treatment IND or parallel track protocols. Decisions by individual states about how to handle these costs through Medicaid will influence physician participation in expanded access protocols; such decisions could determine the level of care provided for impoverished AIDS patients across the country.

Medicare

At present, Medicare does not cover investigational drugs other than Group C cancer drugs, although there is some possibility that this situation may change in the near future.   HCFA is in the process of establishing regulations to govern the Medicare coverage process.   A HCFA spokesman says that when the notice of proposed rulemaking was published in the *Federal Register*, the agency received numerous letters from the public urging Medicare coverage of treatment INDs.   The impact of these letters will not be known until the final rule has been published.

RESOURCES FOR CLINICAL INVESTIGATION

In 1988, the National Institutes of Health (NIH) asked the Institute of Medicine to convene a committee to study issues pertaining to support for clinical investigation.   Several of the committee's recommendations dealt specifically with the role of third-party payers in the clinical trials process.   For example, the committee concluded:

> . . . it is wholly inappropriate for third party payers to deny reimbursement for all appropriate and necessary patient care costs (not marginal costs owing to investigational intervention) that would have been incurred in any case simply because a patient is on an investigational protocol.   Such denial would be tantamount to an abrogation of a contractual obligation. Medicare regulations already will not pay for care of Medicare beneficiaries for investigational therapies that may be the best available treatment.   These policies interfere with the patient-doctor relationship and patient free choice.[2]

The committee also recognized that there are diseases for which appropriate and required care involves investigational protocols.   In

---

[2]Institute of Medicine, *Resources for Clinical Investigation* (Washington, D.C.: National Academy Press, 1988, p. 7).

these cases, the committee said, third-party payers should pay the standard patient care costs while costs related to investigational conclusions should be borne by the drug sponsor—a pharmaceutical company, NIH, or a foundation.

7

IMPROVING ACCESS TO CARE

The previous chapters in this report focused on mechanisms for expanding access to investigational drugs. This chapter addresses a related but slightly different issue: the role of clinical trials and expanded access programs in improving access to health care for the disenfranchised populations that make up the fastest-growing segment of the AIDS epidemic.

By the end of the 1980s it became clear that the demography of the AIDS epidemic was shifting: the rate of new HIV infections among homosexual and bisexual men in major urban centers appears to have dropped. A comparison of AIDS cases reported to the Centers for Disease Control before 1985 and those reported during the first six months of 1989 shows an 11 percent decrease in the proportion attributed to homosexual behavior. In contrast, the proportion attributed to intravenous drug abuse increased by 28 percent. The largest percentage increase—100 percent—occurred among the heterosexual partners and children of intravenous drug abusers.

The men, women, and children at greatest risk of acquiring HIV infection through intravenous drug abuse are among the most disadvantaged members of society. The socioeconomic factors associated with high rates of drug abuse in minority populations are also associated with high rates of HIV infection. Blacks, who make up only 11.6 percent of the U.S. population, account for 27 percent of adult and 52 percent of pediatric AIDS cases. Hispanics, who represent 6.5 percent of Americans, account for 15 percent of adult and 23 percent of pediatric AIDS cases. More than 70 percent of all women with AIDS are black or Hispanic.

This chapter is based on the presentations of Gerald Friedland, Lawrence S. Brown, Jr., Mark Smith, Deborah Cotton, Philip Pizzo, and Harvey Makadon.

Very few of these patients have a regular relationship with a health care provider; as a result, they often lack access to the life-prolonging drugs and services that have become the mainstay of treatment for HIV infection. Some advocates argue that clinical trials and expanded access protocols could be a major avenue for bringing state-of-the-art medical care to this population. (In the past, white males have predominated in almost all clinical trials.) They suggest that including these patients in drug trials would meet several goals: (1) improved medical care for a population that traditionally has been underserved; (2) a more equitable distribution of health care resources; and (3) collection of vital scientific information about the ways in which people of different backgrounds respond to specific investigational drugs.

Other scientists, some with a great deal of experience in providing care to AIDS patients, say that it is not realistic to expect clinical trials or other drug protocols to solve the problem of access to health care. They, too, would like to accomplish the above goals but believe that economic, ethical, and social barriers limit what can be accomplished through drug research.

In fact, some health care providers are concerned that parallel track and other expanded access mechanisms will actually widen the gap in access to medical care between wealthy and indigent populations. Patients who have private physicians with the time and resources to fill out data forms and comply with other requirements of the parallel track will have access to new drugs at the earliest possible moment; patients who do not have primary care providers or who must depend on the overworked staffs of large inner-city hospitals, and those without insurance or other means to pay the costs associated with drug delivery, will be much less likely to gain entry into an expanded access system.

To redress this imbalance, efforts to increase access to investigational drugs must be accompanied by broader measures to improve health care for the entire spectrum of AIDS patients. Ideally, such measures would be incorporated into efforts to improve access to care for all indigent populations in the United States. In the short term, however, AIDS-specific actions must be taken to help states and cities whose health care systems are faltering under the medical and financial burdens of the epidemic.

PEOPLE OF COLOR

Physicians who care for minority AIDS patients list three major barriers to the use of clinical trials as a means of improving access to care for people of color. First, many of the institutions that serve low-income minority patients are already overburdened; they simply are not prepared to follow substantial numbers of patients on new investigational drugs. Second, many people of color view the research establishment and the institutions behind it with suspicion; they may not be willing to participate in programs based at these institutions. Third, the lack of options for impoverished patients raises strong ethical concerns about their ability to give genuine informed consent.

Resource Considerations

Advocates for people with AIDS, government scientists, and physicians all agree that clinical trials should include a more balanced sampling of the population infected with HIV. In the early years of the AIDS epidemic, almost all trials of prospective AIDS drugs involved white gay men. Then scientists became concerned that the results of such trials might not be applicable to the growing population of individuals infected with HIV through intravenous drug abuse, many of whom were people of color. The latter tended to have more concurrent infections, poorer nutrition, and a different natural history of disease—for example, a lower incidence of Kaposi's sarcoma—all of which may alter how drugs work to fight HIV infection. Moreover, clinical trials represented the only access to potentially life-saving drugs; basic considerations of equity argued that they should not be restricted to one patient group.

Increased access for minorities was one rationale behind the Community Programs for Clinical Research on AIDS. In addition, NIAID created a program to support minority medical institutions in developing the necessary operational capabilities for an AIDS clinical trials unit (ACTU) and provided increased funding for existing ACTUs to help them recruit and retain previously underserved populations. The situation is improving. In 1987, only 6.5 percent of the subjects in protocols being run by the NIAID AIDS Clinical Trials Group were black, and 10.6 percent were Hispanic. By 1989, 13.9 percent were black, and 14.1 percent were Hispanic.

Some health care providers say, however, that it may be difficult to progress much beyond these levels. Most of the public hospitals and clinics that serve indigent patients are understaffed and over-crowded. Providing them with funds to conduct clinical trials enables them to hire special research staff, but it does not solve the space problem. In the absence of capital improvements, these institutions might have trouble meeting new expectations.

One of the common goals of community-based trials and expanded access protocols is to enable patients to receive investigational drugs through their own physicians. But many of these physicians are not equipped to determine eligibility for drug trials, to follow and monitor patients on new therapies, and to report on laboratory parameters and adverse reactions. For example, the director of the Boston AIDS Consortium reports that physicians from the city's neighborhood health centers are beginning to attend meetings of the consortium's Clinical Providers Group but that at this time they are more concerned with how to provide basic primary care than with the design and implementation of sophisticated clinical trials. He says:

> Their concerns are about how to keep records confidential; where to get CD4 testing done reliably and at a reasonable cost; how to administer, bill, and get reimbursed for aerosol-ized pentamidine treatments; and how to get their neighbor-hood pharmacies to carry AZT.

> I hope it is clear that if we are to be realistic, the issue of expanding access must be viewed from a broader perspective and has to be considered in the context of our capability to provide primary care generally, our preparedness to provide this for people with HIV infection, and the fact that even when we are doing this, unfortunately, to a great extent, we must weigh competing demands, offering detection, counseling, and initiation of standard antiretroviral therapy versus expanding access to clinical trials.

Programs to place clinical trials in primary care settings often fail to deal effectively with reimbursement issues. New York State has developed enhanced reimbursements for physicians seeing patients with AIDS in designated centers, but this is by no means universal. In most cases, time spent on clinical investigations is added to time spent doing routine care and, often, finding appropriate treatment for patients with drug abuse problems. All of these tasks together may be reimbursed at the same level as a routine office visit. Whatever the means that are finally adopted, government planners must deal effectively with these resource issues to enhance access to investigational drugs through the primary care providers that serve low-income minority patients.

Suspicion

Increasing minority enrollment in clinical trials also depends on greater understanding of the deep ambivalence that exists among people of color with regard to the premier academic research institutions in this country. An AIDS physician from Johns Hopkins University reports that he was greeted with hostility and suspicion when he first attempted to make contact with members of the black community in Baltimore. He discovered that some people growing up in the neighborhoods around the medical center had been told as children that scientists from the medical school snatched black people off the streets at night and put them in the basement to experiment on them. It was clear that the people who told these stories did not believe them in a literal sense, but the fact that they repeated them indicated a general level of unease with the medical establishment.

Individuals in the community also were extremely familiar with the details of the infamous Tuskegee study, in which members of the Public Health Service followed hundreds of poor black men with syphilis for four decades (1932–1972) without offering them treatment. The subjects neither knew nor consented to their role in this "scientifically controlled experiment."

Fears associated with both real and imagined abuses by the research community, combined with persistent memories of segregated care, will continue to hamper recruitment efforts for clinical trials unless they are discussed openly. Too often, there is a tendency to respond with a joke when a patient says, "So you mean I'm going to be a guinea pig, doc?" For people of color—as well as other patients—the question could mask a serious plea for reassurance.

Informed Consent

Reassurance takes on even greater importance for patients who feel they have no alternative to participation in a clinical trial. Chapter 2 explores the difficulties of obtaining genuine informed consent in AIDS-related drug trials. Poor patients may not have the option of forgoing randomization and obtaining a desired drug through some other mechanism.

Some patients also may be at a disadvantage because they do not have the educational skills necessary to understand the complex details of a research protocol.   One way to make protocols more responsive to the needs of such patients is to broaden membership on local institutional review boards (another option discussed in Chapter 2). This would provide a forum for members of the community to educate clinical investigators about the best ways to present new treatment options.

WOMEN

An experienced research nurse at a major academic medical center recently told the principal investigator at her institution that she would much rather see a 40-year-old male engineer in her clinical trials than a young woman with two children who has forgotten the baby's bottle and diapers.   This sentiment illustrates just one of the problems with the expectation that clinical trials could be a major avenue for increasing access to care for women with HIV infection. In most hospitals, the clinics that monitor AIDS drug trials do not have the resources or facilities—in terms of transportation, babysitting services, and staff members knowledgeable about women's health care issues—to meet the needs of women.

The Gender Perspective

In fact, the problems go much deeper than resource issues.   The AIDS epidemic among women differs in almost every respect from the AIDS epidemic among men.   For example, the growth of the epidemic among women is very different.   One scientist suggests that the majority of men who will develop HIV-related illnesses in the next 10 to 20 years are already infected; moreover, a significant proportion have progressed to the symptomatic stages of disease.   In contrast, most HIV-infected women are in the early stages of disease and there is a large population of high-risk women who have yet to become infected.   (This situation has arisen because of the transmission patterns in the United States; early in the epidemic, most transmission occurred through male homosexual activity and intravenous drug abuse—about 70 percent of IV drug abusers are men. Heterosexual transmission did not become a major factor until later.) Physicians who provide health care to women are concerned that too much emphasis on enrolling women in clinical trials could overshadow the tremendous opportunities that still exist for prevention.

Risk Factors

Prevention education and recruitment for clinical trials both require identification of a target population, which raises another difference between men and women with respect to HIV infection. Almost all HIV infection in men is associated with their own personal behavior—either homosexual sex or IV drug abuse. Recent decreases in new infections among gay men and IV drug abusers indicate that educators can reach out to these populations and help them alter the behaviors that place them at risk (for example, by practicing safer sex or "AIDS-safer" injection).

Among women, however, a relatively large percentage of cases occur in individuals with undetermined risk. Many women are infected by sexual partners who have not been truthful about previous high-risk experiences. These women may be completely surprised when they develop symptoms of HIV-related disease or bear an HIV-infected infant.

It is extremely difficult to direct educational efforts toward a population whose members do not realize they are at risk. It is even more difficult to incorporate this population into clinical trials.

Protocol Development

Several drug protocols have been developed recently to study the safety and efficacy of anti-HIV therapy in pregnant women. Although the need for such therapy is clear, protocol development has been problematic for many reasons. First, scientists know very little about the natural history of HIV infection in women in general, and even less about the natural history of the disease in pregnant women. Uncertainty about transmission rates also presents a problem. Several years ago, HIV-infected women were told that they had a 60 percent chance of transmitting the virus to their fetus and that all infected children would die within one to two years. Today, scientists believe that the transmission rate is in the range of 25 to 30 percent and that some infected children will live well beyond their toddler years. But the scientific community still has not determined when in gestation a woman transmits the virus to her fetus. Given these uncertainties, it may be very difficult for a woman to decide whether or not to participate in a clinical trial.

The second problem with recent drug protocols is that they do not take account of the realities of the health care setting. The low-income women who are at greatest risk of HIV infection often have poor prenatal care, late prenatal care, or no prenatal care at all. The expectation that many of them will be identified and enrolled in clinical trials during the first trimester of pregnancy is probably unrealistic.

Women as Vectors

The dominant problem with the protocols for pregnant women, however, is that their major focus is on interrupting perinatal transmission. This reflects a tendency in society to consider women with AIDS only in relation to their ability to transmit infection to their male sex partners or their infants.

One arm of a protocol now in the planning stages would identify HIV-infected women early in pregnancy but not treat them until the onset of labor. Studies in men have shown that early treatment with antiviral agents can delay AIDS-related symptoms, but no one knows the effects of these agents on the developing fetus. Thus, the decision to delay therapy raises very complex issues about the rights of the mother versus the rights of the child.

A New Approach

Efforts to increase access to clinical trials for women will be most successful if they are part of a new gender-specific approach to HIV education and therapy. Such an approach might include greater support for research on the natural history of HIV infection in women, a commitment to include physicians who are knowledgeable about women's health issues in the design of clinical trials, and a unified approach to the scientific, medical, and ethical issues surrounding clinical trials in pregnancy. Women should be viewed as primary recipients of care, and every effort should be made to repudiate the characterization of HIV-infected women as vectors, transmitters, or vessels of disease.

Today, an HIV-infected woman with an infected child is often required to broker her care among four different providers: her routine provider, her clinical trial site, her child's routine provider, and her child's clinical trial site. Even a woman with extraordinary financial and emotional resources would find such a task difficult. For the average woman with HIV infection, who must worry about feeding, clothing, and housing her healthy children as well as her sick children, it is almost impossible. Future efforts to increase access to investigational drugs for women will be most effective in centers that integrate clinical trials with routine medical care for both women and children.

THE PEDIATRIC POPULATION

The AIDS epidemic has produced a dramatic change in the way the scientific community approaches clinical trials in children. In the past, clinical trials were generally not begun in children until safety, and perhaps even efficacy, had been established in adults. The rationale for the delay was that it protected children from exposure to unnecessary experimentation. But the severity of HIV infection and the steady increase in infected children (government officials estimate that the number of HIV-infected children in the United States is between 6,000 and 20,000) have created incentives for change.

Government scientists now recognize the need to begin phase 1 trials in children concurrently with or just slightly after the start of adult trials, which should help avoid the types of problems that arose with zidovudine (AZT). Zidovudine was approved for adults in 1987, but children did not have access to the drug outside of traditional clinical studies until October 1989, when the FDA approved a treatment IND for the pediatric population. Parents and physicians of children with HIV continued to have difficulty obtaining the drug until May 1990, when the FDA waived rules for separate efficacy studies in children and approved the drug for anyone above three months of age.

Over the next few years, clinical trials may play a greater role in pediatric AIDS therapy than in adult therapy, in part because the total number of recognized cases remains relatively small. Also, clinical trials provide a controlled environment in which to begin addressing the scientific and social problems that now impede the delivery of care to children with AIDS.

Scientific Issues

The scientific problems result primarily from lack of experience in conducting clinical trials in newborns and young children and from the paucity of information about the natural history of HIV infection in this age group.   In fact, three-quarters of the drugs that are now part of standard formularies were never tested in children; they are simply used by extension.   Because pharmaceutical companies have very little incentive to produce formulations specifically for the pediatric population, the pace of future clinical trials in children will depend in part on developing such incentives and increasing the availability of appropriate substances.

Scientists also need more information about the progression of HIV-related diseases in children with perinatal infection.   As noted earlier, more HIV-infected children survive infancy than was previously expected, and some children do not develop symptomatic disease until well after their fifth birthday.   Investigators cannot completely assess the efficacy of drug candidates until they understand the factors that determine the onset and pace of disease in the absence of drugs.

Social Issues

Earlier sections have alluded to the fact that most children with perinatal HIV infection come from severely impaired families.   In some cases, the day-to-day demands of poverty and drug abuse may prevent parents from taking an active role in their children's care; in other cases, parents may be severely ill themselves.   Pediatric clinical trials among this population must offer much more than investigational drugs and research-related medical care.   Compliance with trial regimens depends on the availability of a broad range of services to provide physical and emotional support for the entire family.   The multidisciplinary teams developed for pediatric clinical trials could become a model for pediatric AIDS care in other settings.

HIV-infected children who have no family support usually enter the foster care system, a circumstance that raises additional issues. Foster care agencies vary from city to city in their policies on investigational therapies.   The implementation of AIDS-related clinical trials may be difficult in areas where the foster care system does not recognize the importance of access to experimental drugs.

In addition to infants born to high-risk women, one other pediatric population is at great risk of HIV infection: adolescent runaways (officials estimate that there are about a million teenage runaways across the United States).   In large cities, such as New York and San Francisco, runaways often use sex as a way of earning a living, which places them at enormous risk of infection from all types of venereal diseases.   Providing regular health care for these homeless children is extremely difficult; the potential for including them in clinical trials is limited.   The most urgent task with regard to teenage runaways is AIDS prevention education; communications skills developed to help adolescents avoid HIV infection might be used later to promote long-term care for this very challenging target group.